EAR, NOSE AND T

Ear, Nose and Throat Nursing

ANNA M. SERRA
RGN RNT, Senior Tutor, The Royal National Throat,
Nose and Ear Hospital, London

C. M. BAILEY
BSc FRCS, Consultant Otolaryngologist,
The Royal National Throat, Nose and Ear Hospital,
London, and The Hospital for Sick Children, London

P. JACKSON
FRCS FRCSE DLO, Consultant Otolaryngologist,
Lewisham, N. Southwark, and Greenwich and Bromley AHA; formerly,
Senior Lecturer, Institute of Laryngology and Otology, London

BLACKWELL SCIENTIFIC PUBLICATIONS
OXFORD LONDON EDINBURGH
BOSTON PALO ALTO MELBOURNE

© 1986 by
Blackwell Scientific Publications
Editorial offices:
Osney Mead, Oxford, OX2 0EL
8 John Street, London, WC1N 2ES
23 Ainslie Place, Edinburgh, EH3 6AJ
52 Beacon Street, Boston
    Massachusetts 02108, USA
667 Lytton Avenue, Palo Alto
    California 94301, USA
107 Barry Street, Carlton
    Victoria 3053, Australia

First published 1986

Typeset by Acorn Bookwork,
Salisbury, Wiltshire
Printed in Great Britain by
Butler & Tanner Ltd,
Frome and London

DISTRIBUTORS

USA
    Blackwell Mosby Book Distributors
    11830 Westline Industrial Drive
    St Louis, Missouri 63141

Canada
    The C. V. Mosby Company
    5240 Finch Avenue East
    Scarborough, Ontario

Australia
    Blackwell Scientific Publications
        (Australia) Pty Ltd
    107 Barry Street
    Carlton, Victoria 3053

British Library
Cataloguing in Publication Data

Serra, Anna M.
    Ear, nose and throat nursing.
    1. Otolaryngological nursing
    I. Title   II. Bailey, C. M.
    III. Jackson, P.
    617′.51′0024613   RF52.5
    ISBN 0-632-00826-1

Contents

PART III · THE THROAT

Preface

It is now about 10 years since the Joint Board of Clinical Nursing Studies (now incorporated in the English National Board for Nursing, Midwifery and Health Visiting) produced the outline curricula for the ear, nose and throat nursing courses. During this time several excellent books on the speciality have been written but no single text has adequately covered the syllabus as this has not been their intention. The aim of this book is to fill this gap. The authors also hope that basic learners and qualified nurses working in ear, nose and throat areas, as well as those undertaking post-basic training, will find it useful. Although medical practitioners are not the group for which it has been written we also feel that general practitioners and newly qualified doctors will find it helpful when caring for patients with ear, nose and throat disorders.

The authors would like to thank Dinah Taylor and Wendy Ellison for their help with typing the manuscript, and the Department of Clinical Photography, the Institute of Laryngology and Otology, London for their help with the illustrations. Thanks are also extended to Duphar Laboratories Limited, Shiley, for permission to reproduce their photographs. Anna Serra would also particularly like to thank the many nurses who have done (and are yet to do) training in the speciality. They have provided the stimulus for this book, and it is for them that it has been written.

1 Nursing Objectives

Ear, nose and throat nursing is challenging because it involves the care of patients of all ages with a wide variety of conditions of all degrees and severity. In these days of early mobilization and discharge many patients only spend a few days in hospital, although those suffering from more severe disease may be there for several weeks. For many nurses these variations give a balance which they find satisfying.

Having a patient in hospital for only a few days does not exclude the need to take a nursing history, identify nursing problems and plan action to reduce or alleviate these problems. Having set goals the nurse must then evaluate whether or not these have been achieved. A reduction in length of stay does not mean a reduction in the quality of individual patient care.

PRE-OPERATIVE NURSING CARE

The majority of patients in an ear nose and throat ward have been admitted as planned admissions from a waiting list. Knowing the date and time of an operation does not make it any less frightening an experience than an emergency operation. Some might say that it gives the patient more time to think about what is going to happen and what can possibly go wrong. Neither does having the same or a similar operation performed several times make a hospital stay an experience free from anxiety. The nurse should therefore look upon each admission as a new experience for the patient. Never assume that the patient is familiar with what is going to happen during his stay until you have actually been given this information by a patient. There is no such thing as a minor operation to the person involved. Less major it may be, but minor it *never* is. Giving adequate information and psychological prep-

1

aration prior to surgery can aid recovery and reduce postoperative pain and anxiety.

There is a real danger of pre-operative preparation becoming routine to nurses working on an ENT ward unless they constantly remind themselves that to each person the surgery for which he is being prepared is a unique and worrying experience. Each person in the nurse's care is an individual, and care must be planned to meet his particular needs.

General Anaesthetic

In Britain, most ear, nose and throat surgery is performed under general anaesthesia. The following pattern of preparation and care applies to all such surgery. The patient will need to:

1 Have signed a consent form, after being seen by the doctor and before the premedication is given.

2 Fast for at least 4 hours to reduce the risk of vomiting and inhaling gastric contents under general anaesthesia. However, small children become ketotic if starved for much longer than this, an important factor when planning an operating list.

3 Have clean skin, nails and hair to reduce infection and minimize avoidable contamination of theatre.

4 Wear special clothing which is clean, to reduce the risk of infection, and of a style which will aid correct positioning and attachment of equipment in theatre.

5 Remove all prostheses, not forgetting dentures. These may become dislodged and cause obstruction, injury or be lost.

6 Remove all cosmetics to allow observation of skin and mucous membrane colour for cyanosis.

7 Remove all jewellery and hair grips to prevent diathermy burns. If a wedding ring is left on it must be covered by tape to prevent loss and diathermy burns.

8 Empty the bladder to reduce the risk of incontinence in theatre, and restlessness during recovery from anaesthesia.

9 Receive any premedication that is ordered at the correct time.

These points need to be explained to the patient. Most hospitals use some form of pre-operative check list which is completed by the nurse responsible for the patient, before giving premedication.

It is essential that vital signs of temperature, pulse and respiration rates, and blood pressure (TRP and BP) be recorded as baselines for postoperative comparison. A specimen of urine is obtained for ward urinalysis so that, for example, glycosuria due to diabetes, or proteinuria due to renal disease is not overlooked. Local preparation of the operative field may also be necessary, for example shaving or the use of a depilatory cream, prior to aural surgery and application of topical vasoconstrictors prior to nasal surgery. Bowel preparation is also necessary if total pharyngo-laryngectomy is planned.

When the premedication is given the nurse must explain to the patient the effects that it will have. The most frequently used drugs are tranquillizers, hypnotics or narcotics, for example Omnopon or pethidine, which make the patient feel relaxed and sleepy, plus an acetylcholine antagonistic or anticholinergic drug, for example atropine or hyoscine, which will reduce bronchial and salivary secretions and block vagal inhibition of the heart.

Following premedication the patient should not get out of bed as he may be unsteady and fall over. A call bell should always be on hand. There is no reason why a patient should not listen to quiet music or read a book if this is going to help relaxation. Whether screens are totally or partially pulled round the bed varies according to the wishes of the individual ward sister or charge nurse.

If the patient has a tracheostomy or laryngectomy tube *in situ* then a sterile spare tube and introducer of the same style and size should accompany him to theatre.

A visit by a member of staff from the operating theatre and intensive therapy unit to describe what is going to happen to the patient in these departments can do much to relieve anxiety.

The procedure used for checking the patient's identity before leaving the ward and on arrival at the operating theatre *must* be carried out fully on both occasions.

Local Anaesthetic

When the operation is performed using a local anaesthetic the procedure is the same as for a general anaesthetic except that the patient is not required to fast. The premedication ordered will not include an anticholinergic drug, but narcotics, for example Omnopon, not only reduce sensitivity to pain but allay apprehension and anxiety.

General Pre-operative Objectives

1 To obtain sufficient information about the patient to be able to identify nursing problems and plan effective care.

2 To give the patient and his family adequate information about ward routine and pre-operative and postoperative events.
3 To provide adequate physical and psychological support for the patient and his family.
4 To prepare the patient physically and emotionally for a general or local anaesthetic.
5 To ensure that all necessary investigations have been performed, including the sickle-cell test when applicable, and that the results are available.

Specific Objectives Prior to Ear Surgery

1 Identify possible problems in communication and plan nursing actions to solve these. For example, if the patient has a hearing aid, is it working properly and how soon after surgery can it be used? How much hearing is there in the ear which is not going to be operated on? Does the patient depend on lip-reading for communication?
2 Ensure that the patient is aware of any pressure bandage or pack which is to be applied at the time of operation, the reasons for these dressings being used and the approximate length of time that they will be in place.
3 Ensure the patient is aware of the effects of vertigo and nausea if these are a possibility. Explain at this stage how these effects can be minimized by not moving the head quickly and by the use of medication.
4 If pressure change situations, for example flying or travelling by underground trains, are to be avoided during the convalescence period, confirm that the patient is aware of the need and reason for this.
5 Remove hair, by shaving or use of a depilatory cream, from the site planned for incision. The amount of hair to be removed varies according to the site of incision and the wishes of the surgeon. There are three commonly used incisions.

(a) *Postaural* The incision is made over the mastoid bone, behind the pinna. Most surgeons require 2–4 cm of hair to be removed from this area.
(b) *Endaural* The incision is made into the tissues in front of the upper pinna and passes backwards into the outer part of the auditory meatus. Approximately 2–4 cm of hair needs to be removed from the ear just above and in front of the pinna.

(c) *Endomeatal or Permeatal* The incision is made in the posterior skin of the external auditory meatus. To see the incision it is necessary to examine the meatus with the aid of instruments and a light source. It cannot be seen from the outside. It is rarely necessary to remove any hair when this approach is used.

Local skin preparation is usually carried out in the operating department immediately prior to surgery.

Specific Objectives Prior to Nasal and Sinus Surgery

1 If there is to be local preparation of the area, for example by nasal packing or by Moffett's method (see Chapter 6), explain the procedure.

2 Ensure that the patient is aware of the possibility of nasal packs or splints being inserted in the operating theatre. Give an approximate length of time that these packs are to be *in situ* and some indication of the problems that they can cause such as mouth-breathing and loss of smell.

3 Ensure that the patient is aware of the likelihood of post-operative nasal obstruction. Nasal surgery is frequently performed to remove nasal obstruction. The nasal airways will be swollen for varying lengths of time after the surgery, and full resolution may take up to 6 weeks.

4 If a Caldwell-Luc operation or approach is to be undertaken check whether the patient has a dental plate which may encroach upon the incision area, that is, the canine fossa. Swelling and discomfort may prevent such plates from being worn during the immediate postoperative period.

Specific Objectives Prior to Throat Surgery

1 Ensure that the patient and his family are aware of any restrictions on voice use after surgery. Identify possible communication problems and plan nursing action to minimize these.

2 Ensure that the patient and his family are aware of any restriction on fluid and food intake following surgery. If intravenous or tube feeding is planned for the postoperative period the reasons for this and the expected duration must be explained.

3 Ensure that the patient is aware of any incision to be made and any dressings and drains which may be required during the

postoperative period; previous examinations and investigations may have been done by endoscopy which does not require an incision.

Care of a child prior to tonsillectomy and care prior to laryngectomy and tracheostomy are described in the relevant chapter.

POSTOPERATIVE NURSING CARE

Postoperative management of the patient carries the same danger as pre-operative preparation in that if care is not taken one can allow oneself to see the management as routine. This is especially likely to happen in an ENT ward where there may be several patients having the same operation each week. The stereotyping of patients according to the operation that they have had performed will depersonalize the care that is given e.g. the patient is expected to fit into a set pattern of postoperative recovery and achievement, and those who do not may be labelled as difficult or attention-seeking. This way of thinking and caring should be avoided and each patient must be cared for as an individual and care planned according to specific needs.

Pain

It has been said that patients having ENT surgery do not experience much pain! The only person who knows where the pain is and what it feels like is the patient, that is, the person suffering from the pain. Although doctors prescribe analgesics and sedatives it is the nursing staff who have control over administering these drugs as almost all are prescribed to be given as necessary. It is unrealistic to expect every person who has a particular operation to require the same amount of analgesic. Some form of pain relief will be required after almost every surgical procedure and it should be given according to individual needs. The anxious patient is the one most likely to be unable to tolerate discomfort or pain.

Haemorrhage

Following ENT surgery, haemorrhage is often detected by the observant nurse before there is any significant change in vital signs. There are very few places within the area where blood can collect in large amounts before causing swelling or becoming visible to the naked eye. There is always the possibility, however, of blood being swallowed or inhaled and this too should alert the observant nurse.

General Postoperative Objectives

1 To ensure the patient's complete recovery from anaesthesia and ability to maintain adequate ventilation by correct positioning and constant assessment of respiratory function.

2 To monitor vital signs and observe for shock and haemorrhage.

3 To promote wound healing and prevent wound infection.

4 To maintain adequate hydration, electrolyte balance and nutrition.

5 To relieve discomfort and pain.

6 To ensure that the patient's personal cleanliness and comfort is maintained.

7 To ensure that the patient has adequate rest and sleep.

8 To prevent the complications of surgery and bed rest, including deep vein thrombosis, chest infections, pressure area damage and difficulty with micturition or defaecation.

9 To ensure that the patient and his family, have adequate knowledge and understanding of the surgery and care.

10 To give adequate support and teaching to enable the patient to live as normal and independent a life as possible.

11 To ensure that the patient, and his family have sufficient knowledge about continuing care when discharge is imminent.

12 To guide and support the patient towards accepting his altered body and self image when surgery has been disfiguring.

13 To test for glycosuria and ketonuria following head and neck surgery: stress diabetes is a possible complication.

Specific Objectives Following Surgery to the Ear

1 To help the patient maintain a position which will minimize pain and enhance healing.

2 To observe dressings and/or bandages for haemorrhage, and to ensure that they are neither too tight nor too slack.

3 To do regular checks on the function of the VII cranial nerve (facial nerve).

4 To maintain effective nurse/patient communication and re-

lationships. Help the patient reinsert any hearing aid as soon as possible.
5   Observe for nystagmus and vertigo. When vertigo is present, assist the patient in overcoming its effects.

Specific Objectives Following Surgery to the Nose and Sinuses

1   To help the patient maintain a position which will aid drainage, reduce venous congestion and be comfortable.
2   To prevent problems occurring from the presence of anterior and posterior nasal packs. Hypoxia and hypercarbia due to hypoventilation as a result of airway obstruction can occur.
3   To apply measures which will help reduce nasal obstruction and crust formation.
4   To reduce facial oedema.
5   To teach the patient the care of any prosthesis which has been inserted.

Specific Objectives Following Surgery to the Throat

1   Ensure complete return of the swallowing reflex before giving oral fluids or solids.
2   Ensure the absence of trauma which would contraindicate the taking of fluids or solids by mouth.
3   Observe for signs of trauma to the respiratory tract which may gradually lead to respiratory obstruction.
4   Help the patient maintain a position which will prevent inhalation of blood should haemorrhage occur.
5   Make regular and frequent observations of any tracheostomy tube to ensure that it is in the correct position.
6   To help the patient maintain effective communication when the ability to speak is lost.

THE OUTPATIENT DEPARTMENT (OPD)

The outpatient department is frequently very busy as many people who are suffering from ear, nose and throat disorders can be managed as outpatients.

This department has been described as the 'shop window' of a hospital. For most people it is their introduction to the hospital, and as first impressions are usually lasting it is important that the reception and care that is given is of a high standard.

Assisting the doctor during the clinic sessions is only one aspect of the nurse's role in the OPD. The large number of patients passing through the clinic may make it impossible for the doctor to give each patient all the information needed. Alternatively, patients may not fully understand what they have been told, especially if they are anxious or have a hearing loss. In these instances the nurse must make sure that patients have adequate information and knowledge by discussing specific points with them after they have been seen by the doctor. Small booklets outlining the most typical features of a disease and its treatment can be a useful tool in supplementing explanations given in the OPD. These can be very helpful to the patient and his family as the contents can be read at leisure and the booklet kept for future reference. Booklets dealing with conditions such as chronic sinusitis, allergic rhinitis, tonsillitis, deafness in the elderly and glue ear (which account for a fair proportion of OPD appointments) will result in larger numbers of better informed patients.

There are specialist manual skills for the nurse to learn, for example, ear syringing and aural toilet (see Chapter 6). Good communication skills are as essential in this area of nursing as in any other. Many of the patients attending will have a hearing loss. The smooth running of an OPD relies on the management skills of the nursing staff as much as the abilities of the medical and clerical staff. The majority of people attending the clinic will have planned appointments, but emergencies, for example foreign bodies, epistaxis and facial trauma, may result in a patient being referred from an accident and emergency department whilst a clinic is being held.

Most OPD areas have a small 'operating' or treatment room where procedures such as antral washout and nasal polypectomy are performed, with the assistance of the nursing staff, under local anaesthesia. Also considered as part of the nurse's role in many clinics is skin testing for allergic substances on those patients suffering from allergic rhinitis.

General Objectives

1 Make patients and those people attending with them feel welcome.
2 Establish a personal relationship with the patient.

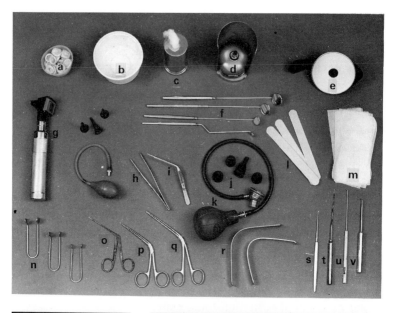

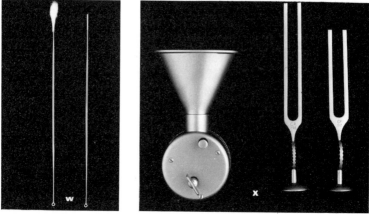

Fig. 1.1 Instruments and equipment found on an ENT examination table.
(a) Finger cots; (b) denture receiver; (c) cotton wool in holder (only the finest grade
wool which is free of small hard pieces is used); (d) spirit lamp; (e) head mirror;
(f) laryngeal and nasopharyngeal mirrors; (g) Welch Alleyn otoscope with specula
and pneumatic attachment; (h) non-toothed dissecting forceps; (i) Keen's aural
dressing forceps; (j) Peter's aural speculae; (k) Siegle's pneumatic attachment;
(l) wooden spatulae; (m) tongue holding swabs (firmly woven smooth swabs);
(n) Thudichum's nasal speculae; (o) crocodile forceps; (p) Tilley's aural forceps;
(q) Tilley's nasal forceps; (r) Lack's tongue depressors; (s) Zanfeld foreign body hook;
(t) Heath's malleable probe; (u) St Bart's blunt hook; (v) Cawthorne wax hook.

3 Ensure that the patient has adequate privacy when describing his problem and during any examination that is performed.

4 Ensure that the patient understands how to:

(a) Take or use any medications prescribed, for example nose drops.

(b) Follow instructions given regarding care, for example how to keep an ear dry whilst washing the hair.

(c) Find the Audiometry, X-ray and Speech Therapy departments as necessary.

(d) Make another appointment.

5 Ensure that the patient has adequate knowledge of his condition and the treatments given.

6 Ensure that the patient has some understanding of any operation which is planned, including the approximate length of hospital stay and length of expected absence from work or school following discharge.

7 Give mental and physical care to the patient, and assist the doctor during investigation such as caloric testing or operations being performed under local anaesthesia.

8 If cocaine has been applied, observe the patient for toxic reactions (see Chapter 6).

9 Assist the doctor during the clinic session, ensuring in particular that there is an adequate supply of instruments and equipment (Fig. 1.1).

10 Ensure that all equipment is kept in good working order and is properly stored.

THE OPERATING THEATRE

It is unlikely that a nurse will achieve more than a general appreciation of the work done in this department during basic or post basic ENT training; more experience is needed to become a skilled theatre nurse.

(w) The Jobson Horne probe is frequently used in the OPD. The circular end is used for removing wax; the other end is serrated and is used as a wool carrier for mopping away secretions and debris. The cotton wool is firmly wound around the serrated end and fluffed out over the end so that the end does not come into contact with tissue. At least six of these probes are needed on an examination tray. (x) A Barany noise box with 256 Hz and 512 Hz tuning forks.

What *can* be gained are the general principles that exist in all operating theatres, for example, safety precautions, gowning and gloving techniques, assisting the anaesthetist, aseptic technique during procedures and the overall care of the patient.

Much of the work is done using an operating microscope which has a teaching arm extension or closed circuit television monitor so that an observer can see the procedure being performed in detail. This is of considerable benefit in understanding the operation and learning the anatomy of the various parts. Knowledge of surgical techniques increases understanding of pre-operative preparation and postoperative nursing problems.

The nose and throat are part of the respiratory tract and the recovery period following investigation or surgery in this area is a potentially hazardous time. Respiratory obstruction is always a danger during recovery from general anaesthesia. It is further complicated following nasal and throat surgery by the danger of inhalation of blood and the nurse must be able to recognize and deal with these emergencies.

PART I · THE EAR

2   Applied Anatomy of the Ear

SKULL

It is impossible to study the skull satisfactorily from a book; one must study the specimen, identifying the named bones and orifices with a teacher or from diagrams (Figs 2.1 and 2.2). It helps to consider the skull in two parts.

The Facial Skeleton

The facial skeleton which makes up about one-third of the skull, is largely a complicated arrangement of thin plates of bone below which hangs the sturdy lower jaw (mandible).

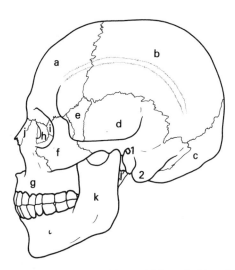

Fig. 2.1   Lateral view of skull. Named bones (a) frontal; (b) parietal; (c) occipital; (d) temporal; (e) sphenoid; (f) zygoma; (g) maxilla; (h) lacrimal; (i) ethmoid; (j) nasal; (k) mandible; (l) styloid process.
   (1) External auditory meatus; (2) mastoid process (part of the temporal bone).

15

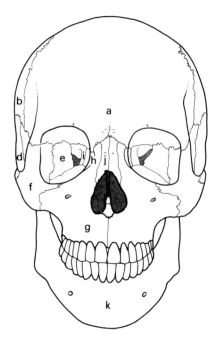

Fig. 2.2   Frontal view of skull. Named bones (a) frontal; (b) parietal; (d) temporal; (e) sphenoid; (f) zygoma; (g) maxilla; (h) lacrimal; (i) ethmoid; (j) nasal; (k) mandible.

The Cranium

The cranium lies above and behind the face. It contains and protects the brain and is composed of stronger bone. The delicate organ of hearing is housed in the petrous part of the temporal bone, a dense bone of the cranium.

OUTER EAR

The conspicuous part seen on the side of the head is the *pinna* or auricle (Fig. 2.3). This is a convoluted sheet of elastic cartilage covered by skin which is closely adherent to it on the outer aspect where the folds of the underlying cartilage are clearly defined. The cartilage is held to the skull by small muscles which in man give the pinna only slight mobility but which contract in response to sound.

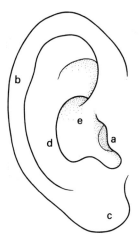

Fig. 2.3 Right pinna (or auricle). (a) tragus; (b) helix; (c) lobule; (d) antihelix; (e) concha.

The pinna of the male carries short hairs, especially on the tragus. The well of the ear leads to the *external auditory canal* or meatus, which is cartilaginous in its outer part. In the adult this is 2.5 cm long, slightly curved, leading medially downwards and forwards (Fig. 2.4). In front of the external canal is the *temporomandibular joint*, and the head of the *mandible* can be felt by the tip of a finger placed in the external meatus on opening and closing the mouth. The skin of the outer half of the canal covers cartilage which is continuous with that of the pinna. The skin here is thick and contains hair follicles and ceruminous glands which secrete wax. The hairs become coarse with advancing years so that retention of wax in the ears is particularly a problem of the elderly. The bony part of the canal is lined with very thin skin (0.2 mm)—this part is short in the infant. At the end of the canal is the *tympanic membrane* (TM) set obliquely so that the posterior part is more accessible than the anterior; indeed the anterior part is often not visible on otoscopy, being concealed in the *anterior recess* formed by the curvature of the bony meatus (Fig. 2.4).

The tympanic membrane (a disc of 1 cm diameter) is normally thin (0.3 mm) and translucent—it has three layers, outer middle and inner (Fig. 2.5). Experimentally, by staining the *outer epithelial layer*, it can be seen that there is a slow migration of this sheet of epithelium from the centre of the tympanic membrane outward

18   *Chapter 2*

onto the wall of the canal and thence along the walls to the outside, the sheet being continually renewed by epithelial growth. This moving sheet carries secretions and debris with it, thus keeping the canal clean. In the middle of the *fibrous layer* is embedded the handle (long process) of the malleus, which is the outermost of the three ossicles. This layer has a thickened rim, the annular ligament,

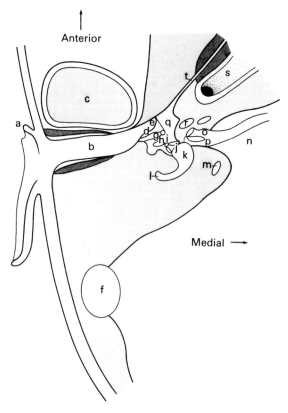

Fig. 2.4   Cross section of the left ear through the Eustachian tube, viewed from above. Semidiagrammatic. (a) Tragus; (b) external auditory canal; (c) head of the mandible; (d) tympanic membrane; (e) anterior recess; (f) sigmoid sinus, carrying venous blood from the brain; (g) malleus; (h) lower end of long process of the incus; (i) head of the stapes, forming a joint with the incus; (j) stapes footplate, closing off the oval window; (k) vestibule; (l) lateral semicircular canal; (m) superior semicircular canal, lying postero-medially; (n) internal auditory meatus; (o) cochlear nerve; (p) vestibular nerve; (q) medial wall of middle ear; (r) cochlea; (s) internal carotid artery; (t) Eustachian tube. The bone surrounding the inner ear structures (l), (m) and (r) is particularly hard and is termed the otic capsule.

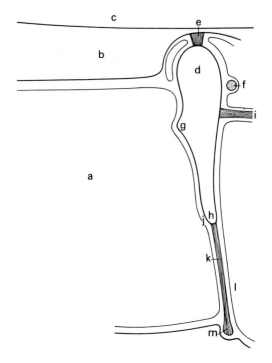

Fig. 2.5 The tympanic membrane. (a) Medial end of the external auditory canal; (b) bony wall of external auditory canal; (c) middle cranial fossa; (d) head of malleus; (e) ligament; (f) chorda tympani; (g) lateral process of malleus; (h) tip of malleus; (i) tendon of tensor tympani muscle; (j) outer layer of tympanic membrane; (k) middle, fibrous layer of tympanic membrane; (l) inner layer of tympanic membrane; (m) annular ligament.

which is held in a corresponding narrow bony groove or sulcus. At operation (e.g. stapedectomy) this ligament can be lifted out of the salcus thus giving access to the middle ear without damaging the tympanic membrane. The *inner layer* is a sheet of flattened epithelial cells continuous with that of the middle ear cavity.

MIDDLE EAR

After birth this cavity (or cleft) within the temporal bone, is filled with air which gains access from the nasopharynx via the *Eustachian tube* as shown in Fig. 2.4. Like the external auditory canal,

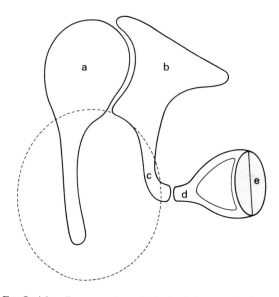

Fig. 2.6 Ear Ossicles, diagrammatic as the body of the incus lies in a plane parallel to that of the TM (dotted line) and the axis of the stapes is at right angles to this. (a) Malleus; (b) body of incus; (c) long process of incus which articulates with (d); (d) head of stapes; (e) stapes footplate.

this tube also lies partly in bone and partly, at its pharyngeal end, surrounded by a plate of cartilage which gives attachment to pharyngeal muscles and is slightly mobile.

At the medial end, the walls of the canal are lightly opposed and the canal is therefore shut; it is opened when the pharyngeal muscles are active, for example on swallowing, yawning or crying. Also, within limits, the canal can be forcibly opened by raising the nasopharyngeal pressure, for example by attempting to blow through the nose whilst it is held closed (Valsalva's manoeuvre).

The lateral part of the Eustachian tube, where it lies in bone, is only 1 mm wide at its narrowest medial end. The cavity of the middle ear is continuous posteriorly with a further cavity, the *mastoid antrum*, and beyond this with a variable interconnected arrangement of air filled spaces in the mastoid bone. The mastoid is said to be 'well pneumatized' if the air cells are extensive—they may be distributed throughout the temporal bone to reach the zygoma anteriorly or the apex of the petrous temporal medially. The mastoid is said to be sclerotic if there are few cells. The *tympanum* is that part of the cavity which lies medial to the

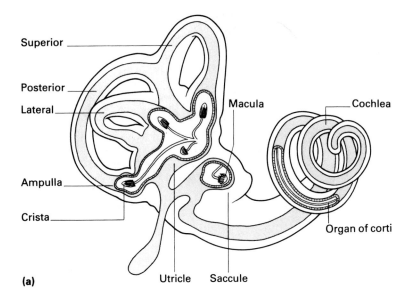

(a)

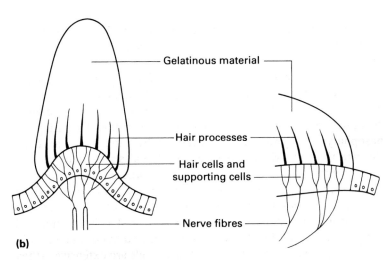

(b)

Fig. 2.7   (a) Diagram illustrating the position of the semicircular canals; utricle and saccule (housing the maculae and cristae); and cochlea. (b) Cross section of the macular (left) and crista where movement of hair processes, as the result of changes in position of the head, stimulate the vestibular nerve fibres carrying information to the brain.

tympanic membrane. This is straddled by the other two ossicles, namely the *incus* and the *stapes*. These three ossicles, the smallest bones in the body, join together to form a chain which transmits vibrations from the tympanic membrane to the inner ear fluid (Fig. 2.6). Delicate folds of mucosa cross the ear to reach the ossicles thus producing several small pockets. In the epithelial lining of the middle ear are scattered areas of ciliated columnar epithelial cells and mucus-producing goblet cells.

INNER EAR

The inner ear contains the sense organs of the VIII cranial nerve: posteriorly, the vestibular system which is concerned with movement and position sense, and anteriorly the cochlea, concerned with the sense of hearing. These parts lie within an inter-communicating system of canals, called the *labyrinth*. The bone surrounding these parts is the dense, *otic capsule* (Fig. 2.4). The labyrinth is lined with a single sheet of flattened cells. Within this bony labyrinth is a similarly convoluted membranous labyrinth which contains *endolymphatic fluid* bathing the sensitive nerve endings of the two systems. Between the membranous labyrinth and the walls of the surrounding bony labyrinth is another fluid of different composition called *perilymph* which communicates via the cochlear duct with the cerebrospinal fluid.

The vestibular system is made up of the three semicircular canals, the utricle and the saccule (Fig. 2.7). The canals are in planes almost at right angles to each other and are named superior, posterior and lateral (or horizontal). The lateral canal is in a vertical plane when a patient lies down with his head 30° above the horizontal plane (see Chapter 5, caloric test); of the three canals, it lies closest to the middle ear. Anteriorly, each canal widens out at the ampulla where there is a patch of sensory epithelium. Similar patches are present in the utricle and saccule.

The cochlea is shaped like a snail's shell with $2\frac{1}{2}$ turns. It is tiny having an overall diameter of about 7 mm. A cross section is seen in Fig. 2.8. The perilymph in the scala tympani becomes continuous with that in the scala vestibuli at the extreme tip of the coil—the helicotrema. Sound vibrations reach the perilymph via the oval window, a defect in the wall of the bony labyrinth closed by the stapes footplate (Fig. 2.8). The round window is a second

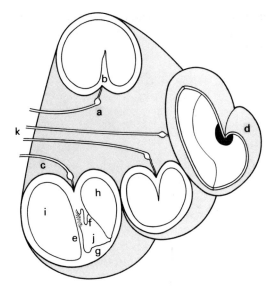

Fig. 2.8 Cochlea (diagrammatic cross section). (a) Central bony pillar (modiolus); (b) bony spiral lamina; (c) basal turn; (d) apical turn; (e) basilar membrane; (f) tectorial membrane; (g) stria vascularis; (h) scala vestibuli; (i) scala tympani (containing perilymph); (j) cochlear duct (scala media); (k) internal auditory meatus.

defect closed by a thin membrane which permits slight oscillatory movements of the labyrinthine fluids. The sensory epithelium bathed in endolymph, lies on the basilar membrane in a spiral strip from the basal turn near the round window to the apex at the helicotrema.

The VIII cranial nerve reaches the cochlea and vestibule via the internal auditory canal. In this canal also runs the VII (facial) nerve which takes a complicated course through the temporal bone where it gives not only the chorda tympani branch, but also a branch to the lacrimal gland and to the stapedius muscle.

3   Clinical Assessment of the Ear

PATIENT HISTORY

The symptoms of ear disease include pain (otalgia); discharge (otorrhoea); dizziness (vertigo); deafness and tinnitus. If these are not all mentioned by the patient it is generally wise to specifically ask about each of them and their duration.

EXAMINATION

Use of the Head Mirror (Fig. 3.1)

This is a skill which nurses specializing in ear, nose and throat are required to master as the equipment has uses other than for examination. It provides a light source and, as both hands are free, it is useful for procedures such as nasal or aural toilet and for the cleaning of a cavity, for example after maxillectomy.

The head mirror is a circular concave mirror with a central hole and a focal length of 18 cm. It is attached to a headband by an adjustable joint.

Friction at the bearing of the mirror to the headband should be such as to allow the mirror to be moved easily and yet stay in the required position. The light from a bull's eye lamp is directed over the patient's left shoulder onto the head mirror. The mirror should then be positioned so that the central hole is close to the examiner's eye, generally the right eye. The patient's head is moved into the beam of light and he can be turned as appropriate; this is facilitated if he sits on a chair or stool that can be rotated. This arrangement allows the examiner the use of two hands, the left one holding an inspecting instrument, for example an aural or nasal speculum or a tongue depressor, and the right hand holding a

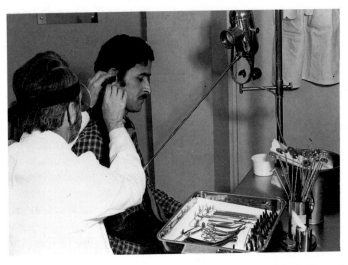

Fig. 3.1   Use of the head mirror in the examination of the ear. (The bull's eye lamp appears to be inactive because of the use of the 'flash' in taking the photograph.) Note the arm on the lamp to facilitate directing the beam of light. The instruments lie conveniently to hand.

mirror for nasopharyngeal or laryngeal examination, or a probe. The table of instruments is generally to the examiner's right for easy access to his right hand. If the right arm interrupts the beam of light it may be helpful to reverse the customary position and have the light directed over the patient's right shoulder.

Appearance

The pinna is examined using a head mirror, noting any abnormalities in shape or position, adjacent scars and conditions of the skin. The external canal and tympanic membrane are inspected by straightening out the lateral cartilaginous part of the canal by gently pulling the pinna in a postero-lateral direction. In children, and sometimes in adults, a good view of the tympanic membrane can be obtained using a well directed mirror without further instrumentation, but generally a better view is obtained using a speculum gently inserted to push aside the hairs and soft tissue of the canal. With practice it is easy to hold the speculum with the index finger and thumb and draw out the pinna with the remaining fingers, the index finger assisting (Fig. 3.1). This allows the other hand to hold a probe or hook or the bulb of a Siegle speculum. The Siegle speculum allows air to be gently blown into the external auditory canal so that the mobility of the tympanic membrane can be seen. The lens in the speculum gives useful magnification—it is at an angle to the axis of the speculum so that the dazzle of reflected light from the lens' surface does not obscure the view.

Inspection, especially if there is middle ear disease, is generally more satisfactory if an electric otoscope is used. The instrument should be held like a pen rather than in the palm of the hand, giving better control as the hand holding the instrument is in contact with the patient's cheek. Otoscopes hitherto generally available have had disappointing optical and lighting arrangements; the speculum has to make a firm fit and with a metal speculum the slightest distortion prevents it seating properly in the instrument. Even with the speculum properly mounted and then inserted as far into the canal as it will go, the focal plane is often lateral to the tympanic membrane so that an enlarged, but blurred, view is obtained. Some otoscopes have a small movable lens to allow instruments to be passed into the speculum and used under magnification, but as generally one still needs to use a second hand to retract the pinna there is not a hand available to use another

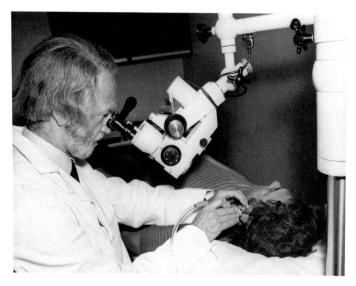

Fig. 3.2 Toilet of the ear using the operating microscope. Note the teaching arm extension from the eyepiece.

instrument—cleaning the ear canal while using a head mirror is easier.

An otoscope is now available with fibreoptic lighting, black plastic specula and a good optical system. A side-arm and bulb are available for 'siegleisation'. Even if there is wax in the canal, such a good view can be obtained with this otoscope that it is often possible to use a very small speculum and manoeuvre it around the obstruction if space permits.

Undoubtedly the best method, though it takes time and it is only worthwhile in difficult cases or where specially indicated, is to use the operating microscope. A well-equipped ENT department should have this facility. Here the patient can lie down with his head supported on a pillow and the examiner can sit comfortably at his work. This allows for suction and accurate toilet (Fig. 3.2).

The examiner must be familiar with the appearance of the normal tympanic membrane (Fig. 3.3) before he can appreciate and interpret abnormal findings. In order to interpret what he sees, he should look for landmarks working from the more certain to the less certain. To learn the normal appearance, follow the posterior meatal wall medially and forwards. This ends at the annulus, often seen as a firm line marking the margin of the posterior part of the tympanic membrane. This part of the tympanic membrane is translucent, and with good illumination there is the impression that light reflected from the red mucosa of the lining of the middle ear can be seen through the TM. Often the long process of the incus can be seen through the membrane postero-superiorly. Carrying the inspection further forwards superiorly the next landmark is the lateral process of the malleus. This is an obvious and important landmark because in middle ear disease it is rarely destroyed in the absence of previous surgery. It is seen as a prominent white knob. In continuity below this can be seen the handle of the malleus as a whitish streak. This is described as pointing inferiorly and pos-teriorly and is so represented on drawings; but the eye appreciates the obliquity of the tympanic membrane and the posterior inclination (not always obvious). Inferiorly the handle of the malleus ends at the *umbo*.

Below the umbo there is a triangular glistening area of tympanic membrane—the *cone of light* indicated on Fig. 3.3. Because the tympanic membrane is obliquely set and slightly concave, this localized area of the healthy drum is generally the only part perpendicular to the rays of light from the external canal, so light

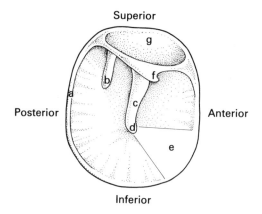

Fig. 3.3 Otoscopic view of right TM. The anterior part of the TM may be obscured by the wall of the canal: (a) annulus; (b) long process of incus, often just visible through the normal TM; (c) handle of malleus; (d) umbo; (e) cone of light; (f) lateral process of malleus; (g) attic.

striking this region is reflected back to the eyes, known as the 'normal light reflex'. The tympanic membrane in front of the umbo in many cases is obscured by the anterior canal wall. Debris may lurk here in the anterior recess. Having identified the landmarks so far it is important next to inspect the *attic*. This lies above the lateral process of the malleus and is easily missed or forgotten, but ear disease may arise here when the remainder of the tympanic membrane looks otherwise normal.

Function

Hearing

The hearing ability is judged in a crude way whilst talking to the patient in taking the history, but of course this will judge the hearing in the better ear. Before audiometry became widely used, quantitative measurement was made by assessing the patient's ability to hear the spoken word from set distances, the ear not under test being occluded. This has little point now, but it is still used as an assessment for disability pension. Many patients who are deaf have acquired a certain facility to lip-read and it is important during the taking of a history when deafness is suspected, to talk to the patient in such a way that he cannot see the examiner's lips. This can easily be done by tactfully holding up the notes across the front of the face between the patient and the examiner or by talking to the patient from behind or when momentarily turned away. This simple trick may surprisingly reveal the patient to be profoundly deaf.

Tuning fork tests are of the utmost importance in making a diagnosis as they are probably the best way of being certain as to whether the patient has conductive or sensorineural hearing loss.

RINNE TEST

The Rinne test compares hearing by bone conduction with hearing by air conduction. The base of a vibrating tuning fork is held firmly on the mastoid bone and the patient is asked to indicate when he can no longer hear it. The fork is then removed and straightway held close to the external canal. If there is no deafness or if there is a sensorineural loss only, the patient can still hear the sound, that is, hearing by air conduction is better than by bone and the Rinne

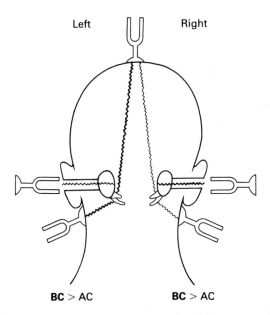

Fig. 3.4 Conductive deafness in the left ear. The left Rinne is negative, and in Weber's test, sound is referred to the left side. (Adapted by kind permission from Foxen, E. H. M. (1980) *Lecture Notes on Diseases of the Ear, Nose and Throat*, 5th edn., p. 11. Blackwell Scientific Publications, Oxford.)

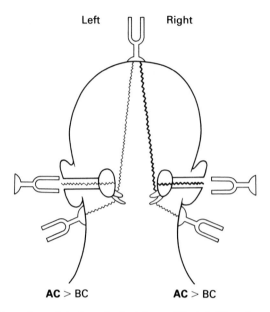

Left   Right

AC > BC   AC > BC

Fig. 3.5 Sensorineural deafness in the left ear. The left Rinne is positive and in Weber's test, sound is referred to the right side. (Adapted by kind permission from Foxen, E. H. M. (1980) *Lecture Notes on Diseases of the Ear, Nose and Throat*, 5th edn., p. 11. Blackwell Scientific Publications, Oxford.)

is said to be 'positive'. If the patient hears better by bone conduction, a 'negative' Rinne, then he has a conductive hearing loss (Figs. 3.4 and 3.5). However, if the ear under test has a profound sensorineural loss then the bone-conducted sound may still be heard, but by the opposite ear, whilst the air-conducted sound is not heard. This simulates a negative Rinne, but if recognized, is recorded as a 'false-negative' Rinne. It is important to be aware of this possibility as such patients may be thought to have a conductive deafness and thus referred for a middle ear operation when no such operation will be helpful. A quicker, but not so reliable assessment can be made by asking the patient to compare simply the loudness of the vibrating tuning fork by air and by bone conduction.

WEBER TEST
In the Weber test a vibrating tuning fork is held against the middle of the skull or on the upper incisor teeth and the patient is asked to point to where he hears it. If the patient has a conductive hearing

loss in one ear he hears it on that side. With a bilateral conductive hearing loss it is heard on the side with the greater degree of conductive loss. With a sensorineural hearing loss the tuning fork seems louder in the better hearing ear (Figs. 3.4 and 3.5). If from the Weber and Rinne tests a false-negative Rinne is suspected, it is worthwhile repeating the Rinne using a Barany box (Fig. 1.1) on the good ear. This instrument makes a loud noise (120 dB) which effectively masks vibrations heard in the good ear by bone conduction from the opposite side.

LOMBARD TEST

Unilateral feigned deafness can be prettily revealed by using the Lombard test. Here when the Barany box is placed over the deaf ear while the patient is reading aloud, there is no difference in the tone of his voice, but when placed over the good ear the patient will raise his voice. If the patient has two good ears but pretends one of them is not good then this raising of the voice is absent.

BING TEST

This test, like the Rinne test, is used to detect a conductive hearing loss. When the vibrating tuning fork is applied to the mastoid bone, the patient with normal hearing in the ear under test hears this louder if the external meatus is occluded, for example by pressing the tragus, but if there is a conductive loss the sound is no louder.

Eustachian Tube

The patency of the Eustachian tube can be tested by the Valsalva's manoeuvre. Here the patient attempts to blow the nose, but with the nostrils pinched. This increases the pressure in the naso-pharynx and normally drives air up the Eustachian tube into the middle ear. In a positive test the outward movement of the intact tympanic membrane can be seen using an otoscope—if the tympanic membrane is perforated, air can be heard to escape from the ear.

Some patients simply do not have the knack of carrying out this manoeuvre, for them and for children it may be worthwhile carrying out Politzerisation (Fig. 3.6). Here a rubber bulb (Politzer's bag) is connected to one nostril, the other being occluded, and the doctor squeezes the bag at the precise moment

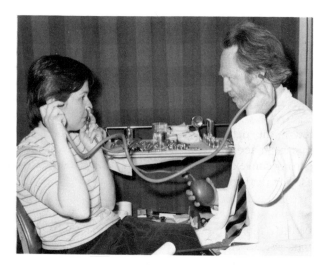

Fig. 3.6 Politzerisation.

when the patient swallows. The swallowing movement closes off the nasopharynx from the oropharynx and opens the lower end of the Eustachian tube. If positive, the resulting movement of air in the middle ear can be heard using a simple connecting tube from the patient's ear to the doctor's ear, but generally the patient will indicate something has happened in the ear, and this is more reliable.

Vestibular System

The patient's gait on entering the consulting room may provide evidence of instability, for example, by touching the wall or making contact with a chair for support. There are further tests which may be performed in the consulting room. In Romberg's test the patient stands erect with the eyes closed and feet together; he will sway or begin to fall if the test is positive. In Unterberger's test the patient 'marks time' with the eyes closed, arms outstretched and hands clasped in front. This is a critical test and if there is no rotation, it is probably true to say there is no cerebellar or vestibular abnormality, though some apparently normal subjects may rotate as much as 90° in 60 seconds. For the other tests, the reader is referred to more specialized texts.

Much of the testing of the vestibular function relies on the nervous connections between the vestibular nuclei and the nuclei controlling eye movement (the occulomotor nuclei). The abnormality one is looking for is nystagmus which consists of a jerky to and fro movement of the eyes. Spontaneous nystagmus should be sought with the subject looking straight ahead and also looking 30° to the right and to the left. Nystagmus due to vestibular disease is enhanced if the patient has nothing on which to fix his gaze. Fixation can be abolished using Frenzel glasses in the dark, these have a strong convex lens and contain an electric light to illuminate the eyes. For further tests, see Vestibulometry, Chapter 5.

Positional nystagmus is revealed by moving the patient, who is sitting on a couch, to a lying position—nystagmus occurs in the new position. If disorder in the neck is thought to be relevant either because of skeletal changes or because of neck posture affecting the blood flow to the posterior part of the brain, then the effect of rotation of the neck in the new position can be assessed. In benign positional nystagmus, the abnormal eye movement commences after a short delay, and the patient becomes very distressed, but it quickly passes off.

4   Physiology of Hearing and Vestibular Function

HEARING FUNCTION

The phenomenon of sound is due to the ear's ability to detect minute rapid changes in pressure, which in turn are due to a disturbance of molecular movement in the air, produced by the source of the sound—sound cannot travel in a vacuum. This disturbance is somewhat analogous to the waves which ripple outwards from a stone thrown into a smooth pond. The change in pressure may be such as to move the centre of the tympanic membrane through a distance of only a fraction of the diameter of a hydrogen atom and yet be heard as sound. If the pressure changes are regular, the ear registers them as a musical note—a pure tone. Such sounds are used in pure tone audiometry, and the human ear can detect sounds from a frequency of about 20 Hz (vibrations per second) to about 20 000 Hz. The upper limit is lower in the elderly.

The outer ear collects the sound. The human pinna has little importance in this connection, but cupping the hand to the ear increases the loudness of ambient sounds. It would seem the main function of the outer ear is to allow the delicate tympanic membrane to be protected at depth in the skull.

The sensory epithelium lies in a fluid medium so that, to be heard, air borne vibrations have to be transmitted to this fluid. Air borne vibrations striking a water surface are reflected by it—only a thousandth of the energy is imparted to the water. This fact accounts both for the silent world of the underwater swimmer, who can only hear sounds generated in the water, and for the hearing loss in glue ear (see Chapter 7).

The function of the middle ear cavity and the ossicles is to 'match' the air borne vibrations to produce vibrations in the inner ear fluid without appreciable loss of energy. The rapid pressure changes (vibrations) of the inner ear fluids are initiated by movement of the stapes footplate. The *basilar membrane* becomes broader as it reaches the apex of the cochlea and this part vibrates maximally when sounds of low frequency reach it. The lower part of the membrane nearest the footplate vibrates to sounds of high frequency so that effectively the energy of the fluid-borne high frequency vibrations is transmitted selectively across this part of the system. The *organ of Corti* (Fig. 4.1), the spiral organ, is located here and is therefore stimulated maximally. This is a simplified account, but essentially the frequency of the vibration determines the pattern of nerve impulses from the spiral organ which in turn is interpreted as the sound heard by the listener. It is thus tiny differences in the linear movement of the inner ear fluids which can be appreciated as speech. The movement of the basilar membrane distorts the organ of Corti and this distortion results in an active metabolic process within the cells resulting in the generation of nerve impulses carried in turn to the brain via the VIII nerve.

VESTIBULAR FUNCTION

The awareness of our position in space is dependent on information from proprioceptors (e.g. pressure receptors in the skin and joints and stretch receptors in muscles), from vision and from the vestibular system of the inner ears. The semicircular canals are in three planes approximately at right angles to each other, and the posterior canal on one side is in a plane parallel to that of the superior canal in the other. The lateral canals are in the same plane.

The hair cells of the ampullae of each canal (Fig. 2.7) are buried in a gelatinous cap which reaches across to the opposite wall. If, for example, the head is rotated in a horizontal direction the ampulla moves, but the movement of the contained fluid lags behind, resulting in displacement of the hair cells. With the head stationary there is a spontaneous resting rate of nerve impulses from the ampulla. Movement in one direction increases this discharge and in the other direction reduces it.

Because of the anatomical arrangement of the lateral canals on each side of the head any horizontal movement (or any movement with a horizontal component) produces an increase in the dis-

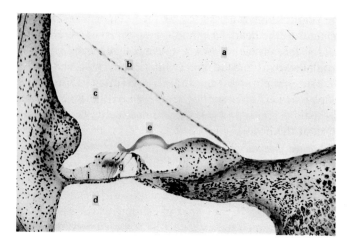

Fig. 4.1 Organ of Corti. (a) Scala vestibuli: contains perilymph and leads into the vestibule; (b) vestibular membrane (also called Reissner's membrane); (c) scala media: contains endolymph; (d) scala tympani: contains perilymph and is continuous at the apex of the cochlea with the scala vestibuli (in the opposite direction it terminates at the round window); (e) tectorial membrane. This is fibrous and acellular; (f) stria vascularis; (g) outer hair cells; (h) inner hair cells and associated supporting cells; (i) basilar membrane; (j) bony spiral lamina. The Organ of Corti is the receptor organ of hearing and consists of one row of inner hair cells and three rows of outer hair cells. The hairs of these calls project into the tectorial membrane. (Reproduced by kind permission of Duphar Laboratories Ltd.)

charge of impulses from one side and a corresponding decrease from the other. The normal sensation of movement depends on the integration of information from both sides—if information from one side conflicts with that from the other, or with information from other proprioceptors, the patient suffers vertigo.

If one is slowly rotated to the right, the natural reaction is for the vision to fix on an object and follow this round for a while; then the eyes are quickly brought back to a mid position and the process repeated. Thus the head and eyes move slowly to the left and a corrective movement is made in the direction of the rotation. This co-ordination of eye and head movement is dependent on a functioning vestibular system with the resulting impulses reaching the centre in the brain for co-ordination of eye movement. The vestibular system and its connections are commonly tested by observing and recording eye movements in response to challenging situations.

The semicircular canal system is thus responsible for detecting *movements* of the head. Information on the *position* of the head is given by the utricle. Here a patch of sensory epithelium is horizontal with the head erect. Suspended in the hairs of the epithelium are two otoliths or 'ear stones'. It appears that the relevant mechanism is simply operated by gravity acting on the otoliths and thus distorting the hairs in a manner depending on the position of the head.

5 Audiometry and Vestibulometry

AUDIOMETRY

Subjective tests

The following tests are 'subjective', that is, they depend on the active voluntary response of the patient.

Pure Tone Audiometry

While clinical examination together with the use of the tuning fork and Barany box may give sufficient information for diagnosis, a more critical examination of hearing acuity is generally required for management. Pure tone audiometry assesses the loudness at which the patient can hear pure tones. Using the audiometer, the technician selects a sound he expects the patient to hear. The patient presses a button (in Fig. 5.1 seen in the patient's right hand) when he hears the sound, releasing it when he no longer hears it. In Fig. 5.1 the test is being carried out with the technician and the patient in the same sound-treated room. A better arrangement is to have the patient in a sound-treated room or booth while the technician and the equipment are outside. The technician should be able to see the patient through a double glazed window and to communicate with him via a microphone and loudspeaker.

The audiometrician adjusts the intensity of the output of the audiometer at each of a number of fixed frequencies, determining the point (threshold) at which the patient indicates he can repeatedly just hear the tone and these are then plotted on a graph.

The intensity is measured in decibels (dB) on a logarithmic scale, an increase of 10 dB measuring a tenfold increase in energy of the sound. The zero level on the audiogram (Fig. 5.2(a))

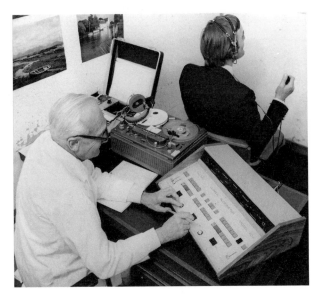

Fig. 5.1 Audiometry. The technician is operating a pure tone audiometer, also on the table are a tape recorder, used for speech audiometry, and an impedance audiometer.

represents the average threshold of hearing of a group of young people who had no history of ear disorder. As it is an average, it follows that some people, generally children, will have a normal hearing level better than average, that is, less than zero. The lower limit of normal is generally accepted as 20 dB. If hearing by air conduction corresponds closely with hearing by bone conduction, the loss is sensorineural not conductive.

Figure 5.2(b) shows a high tone sensorineural hearing loss (SNHL) with a maximum loss at 4000 Hz (4 KHz). Acoustic trauma characteristically causes an initial loss at this frequency which can be detected before there is any noticeable disability. With further exposure to noise there is increasing loss over the neighbouring frequencies and speech discrimination is affected. The tracing for the left ear on this figure shows hearing by bone conduction to be better than air conduction; there is an air-borne gap indicating a conductive hearing loss.

Masking the ear which is not under test (for which the reader is referred to more detailed texts) is important if the audiogram is not to be misleading when carrying out bone conduction audi-

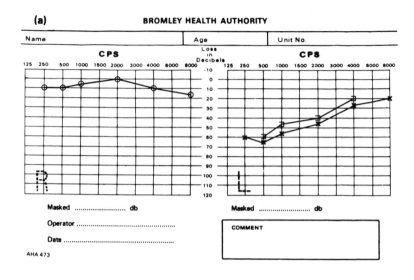

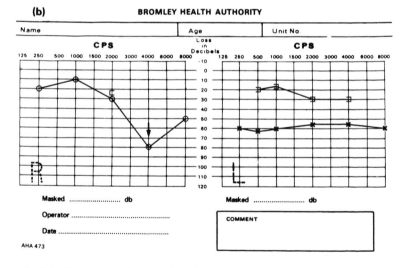

Fig. 5.2 Pure tone audiograms (PTA). Note the symbols used. (a) This tracing shows normal hearing in the right ear; because 0 db is an average, it is exceptional for any individual to give a flat tracing at this level. The tracing for the left ear shows low tone (frequency) hearing loss. Low tone sensorineural hearing loss is a feature of Meniere's disease. (b) High tone SNHL in the right ear. The tracing for the left ear shows a hearing level by air conduction of 60 db; bone conduction is much better and there is an air-borne gap of 45 db over low frequencies. Here deafness is due to conductive hearing loss for example from chronic suppurative otitis media (CSOM). Air conduction: right ○, left ×. Bone conduction: masked right ⊏, left ⊐

ometry. It is also important in determining air conduction thresholds where there is a gross difference in hearing (e.g. >50 dB) between the two ears as otherwise only the better ear will hear the test sound.

Pure tone audiometry can be used to assess the hearing of the co-operative child over the age of 4 years. Between the ages of 2 and 4, there is more co-operation if the response is made into a game rather than the child being expected to press a button. For example the child may put a coloured ball into a basket every time he hears a sound, or add to a stack of bricks. At a younger age, distraction techniques are used in which the attention of the child (who is generally sitting on a parent's lap) is engaged in play while the audiometrician, out of sight behind the child, makes a noise. If the child turns the head in the appropriate direction, he has heard and localized the sound. For the neonate, the startle response is induced if a significant sound has been heard.

Pure tone audiometry requires tact by the audiometrician and perseverance, concentration and patience on the part of the subject. The interested student is advised to undergo pure tone audiometry himself.

Patient Actuated Audiometry

With the recognition that industrial noise causes deafness (noise induced hearing loss, NIHL), monitoring audiometry for workers became important. Sufficient audiometricians are not available and so patient actuated audiometry is increasingly carried out using, for example, a Rudmose machine. The subject is presented with a low pitched sound which increases in frequency and in intensity, producing a continuous tracing on the audiogram. When he hears the sound the subject presses a button which results in the sound becoming quieter; when he no longer hears the sound, he releases the button again. Thus a zigzag trace (Fig. 5.3) is produced. The Bekesy audiometer which is sometimes used in hospital practice gives a similar tracing, but whereas with the Rudmose audiometer a number of fixed frequencies is used, with the Bekesy audiometer the increase in frequency is gradual.

Speech Audiometry

Here the ability of the patient to recognize words on pre-recorded tapes is assessed at various loudness levels and recorded appropri-

42   Chapter 5

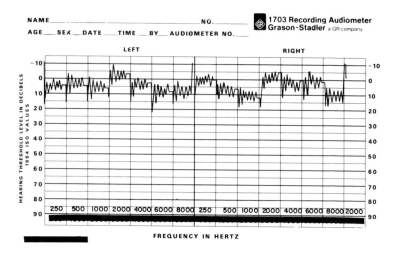

Fig. 5.3 Tracing from a self-actuated audiometer of the Rudmose type. The output is recorded automatically on the graph which shows an oscillating line. In this example the hearing is normal.

NAME: NUMBER:

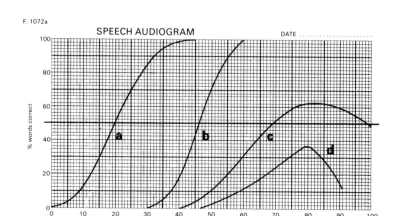

Fig. 5.4 Speech Audiogram. (a) Normal; (b) conductive hearing loss, note the tracing runs approximately parallel to (a); (c) Meniere's disease: may show a number of patterns between (b) and (d), note fall off with increasing amplification; (d) V111 nerve tumour: may also show a number of different patterns, the least affected resembling those of Meniere's disease.

ately (Fig. 5.4). This is important in diagnosis and management. If a good score can be reached with amplification, then surgery or a hearing aid may be helpful. There may be a discrepancy between the speech audiogram and the intelligibility expected from the pure tone audiogram, as in VIII nerve tumour. Alternatively the pattern may be characteristic, showing a fall off in discrimination with increasing amplitude, for example, in Meniere's disease and where there is recruitment.

Objective Tests

The following tests do not depend on the patient's signalling—they are 'objective'.

Electric Response Audiometry

Using appropriate electrodes, electrical activity evoked by sound, in either the cochlea and the adjacent VIII nerve (electrocochleogram, ECochG) or in the more central pathways of the nerve impulses through the brain (auditory brainstem response, ABR), can be detected and displayed. The electrical signals pass through a computer which averages the random background electrical activity. The patterns may be diagnostic of hearing or brain disorders. Because the response is not dependent on the active cooperation of the patient ECochG is invaluable in investigating the hearing of handicapped children who, if restless, can be sedated or even given a general anaesthetic for the test. ABR is playing an increasingly important role in the diagnosis of lesions affecting the VIII nerve (notably acoustic neuroma) and the more central pathways.

Impedance Audiometry

If a sound is made in the external auditory canal, some of the sound energy will be collected by the tympanic membrane whence it is transmitted to the middle ear structures and the perilymph—the rest will escape from the ear after reflection from the walls of the ear canal apart from a small amount which is absorbed by the surrounding tissues. If the external orifice is closed, the energy confined to the space can be measured (Fig. 5.5) and the amount transmitted to the middle ear structures determined. This will be greatest when the tympanic membrane and middle ear structures

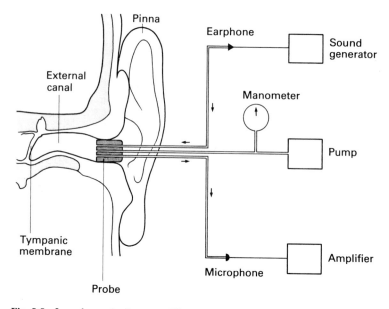

Fig. 5.5 Impedance Audiometry. The generator delivers sound energy into the external canal. The microphone measures the energy in the canal: this is least if the energy has been transmitted efficiently to the middle ear structures. The probe carries the parts as illustrated and it makes a seal in the external canal so that the pressure in the canal can be varied by the air pump.

offer least resistance, or more correctly *impedance*, to the vibrations. Normally this will occur where the ossicles and tympanic membranes are healthy, and the middle ear pressure is atmospheric. This situation is manifest on the tracing as a peak at zero pressure (Fig. 5.6). In carrying out impedance audiometry, the configuration of the tympanic membrane is altered by reducing and increasing the air pressure in the external canal. Similarly, movement imparted to the tympanic membrane by contraction of middle ear muscles, for example in response to a sufficiently loud sound, will change the impedance. Effusion in the middle ear prevents the TM from moving in response to changes in pressure, as in glue ear, and hence the tracing is flat (Fig. 5.6).

Post Auricular Muscle Response Audiometry

This test depends on the reflex contraction of the small post auricular muscles (see Chapter 2) in response to sound signals

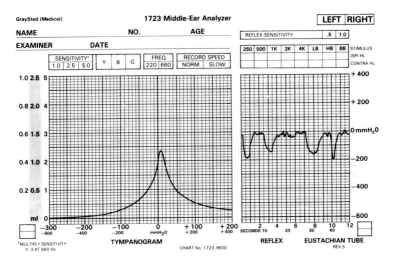

Fig. 5.6 Impedance audiogram. The instrument in most common use nowadays makes an automatic tracing. In the normal subject the middle ear pressure is atmospheric, shown as a peak at zero pressure (left hand tracing). Glue ear (right hand tracing); middle ear effusion prevents movement of the TM in response to changing pressure and the tracing is flat.

reaching the brain. In the test, a series of click sounds is presented to the subject over a period of a few minutes and an electrode behind the ear detects any contraction of the post auricular muscle. The responses are fed into a computer and a comparison is made between the number of clicks and the number of responses. By using clicks of various intensities a threshold level for the detection of click noises can be determined. Alternatively, it may simply be used as a screening test and is of particular value in child assessment.

VESTIBULOMETRY

We have seen in Chapter 3 that the vestibular system and its connections are generally assessed by observing and recording eye movements in response to challenging tests.

There is a potential difference between the front and the back of the eye with the result that movement of the eye will produce changes in electrical potentials which can be recorded by electrodes placed on the adjacent skin (Fig. 5.7). This allows eye

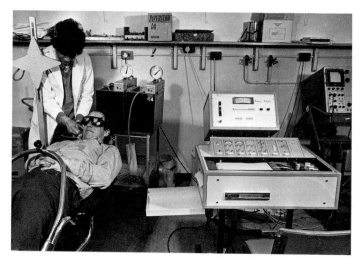

Fig. 5.7 Vestibulometry. The technician is carrying out a caloric test on the patient's right ear.

movement to be recorded when the patient's eyes are closed or when he is in the dark. These conditions enhance nystagmus of vestibular origin, but tend to reduce nystagmus due to cerebellar dysfunction. Using this set up a battery of tests includes recording:

1 Spontaneous nystagmus, both with and without fixation.
2 Positional nystagmus (and 'positioning' nystagmus).
3 Pendulum tracking. The patient watches a pendulum swinging. The normal tracing of the eye movements is a sinusoidal curve.
4 Optokinetic nystagmus. The patient looks at a drum with vertical lines or objects on it, while it is rotated first in one direction and then the other. The nystagmus pattern for one direction of rotation should be a mirror image of the other.
5 Caloric testing (Fig. 5.7). If the horizontal semi-circular canal is made vertical (e.g. by the patient lying on his back with the head flexed 30°) then a convection current of the fluid in the semi-circular canal can be induced by cooling or heating it. This is simply carried out by irrigating the external auditory canal with warm (44°C) or with cold (30°C) water. This unilateral stimulation results normally in profound vertigo and nystagmus. In the standard (Hallpike) technique, the irrigation lasts for 40 seconds. From visual inspection of the eye movement, the criterion of measurement is the duration of the response, normally about 2

minutes, but using electronystagmography the angular velocity of eye movements can be measured and compared. The interpretation of the results lies outside the scope of this book.

This procedure is usually carried out by a member of the medical staff with assistance from a nurse.

Most ENT departments have thermostatically controlled water tanks for caloric testing, otherwise a douche is used. Tanks will need to be filled and switched on at least 30 minutes before the test. To confirm that the thermostat is working properly the water temperatures should be checked with a lotion thermometer. The head of the couch used is raised 30° from the horizontal and it is covered by a mackintosh and towel.

The procedure and possible effects are explained to the patient. He is made comfortable on the pillowless couch; his clothing must be protected. The doctor may wish to inspect the ears and tympanic membranes for wax or perforations before commencing the test.

Most doctors irrigate with water at 44°C first. A stop watch is used to time the duration of the irrigation and subsequent nystagmus. It is important that the watch is started at precisely the same time as the clamp on the caloric tubing is released and irrigation commenced. The nurse may be asked by the doctor to release and clamp the tubing.

The irrigation water is collected in a receiver placed under the ear. A spare receiver should be nearby in case vomiting occurs.

At the end of the test the patient is allowed to recover from any vertigo or nausea. The external auditory canals will need to be dried with cotton-wool dressed applicators.

6 Conditions of the Outer Ear

PINNA

The commonest malformation is the absence of the ear lobe. More noticeable deformities are the 'lop' ear, in which the upper part of the pinna falls downwards, and the 'bat' ear. The function of the ear is normal and deformity can often be ignored or hidden. School children with these deformities (and a short hair style) may be teased mercilessly; correction of the deformity by surgery may be advisable after the age of six when the pinna has virtually ceased growing. This is carried out via an incision on the posterior aspect and skin and cartilage are trimmed as necessary to give an acceptable result.

Nursing Management in Bat Ears

A child old enough to have this deformity corrected can understand and appreciate simple explanations of what is going to happen to him before and after the operation.

No local preparation is necessary other than a thorough examination of the scalp and hair. Presence of head lice or nits will result in the operation being postponed—they are likely to cause wound infection and almost unbearable itching and discomfort.

On completion of the operation the child will have a firm dressing of cotton wool and a crepe bandage applied. An operation on both ears will require a figure of eight bandage. This is necessary to give adequate support to the newly formed pinna. Upon wakening the child becomes aware of his reduced hearing, due to the presence of the dressings. This is a traumatic experience and he will almost certainly try to remove the dressings. It needs skill and understanding on the part of the staff to prevent this, and any analgesics or sedatives ordered should be given.

The stay in hospital is a brief one although the dressings applied remain in place for about 2 weeks. During this time every effort must be made to keep the child happy and occupied. Prior to discharge parents need to be advised about the dangers to a child with reduced hearing, especially when in the street. They should be discouraged from allowing the child out to play on a bicycle beyond the confines of an enclosed garden.

At the end of 2 weeks the child returns to outpatients for removal of the dressings and the bandage. If the surgeon wishes the parent to apply a dressing and bandage to the ears before the child goes to bed each night for a period, the nurse should demonstrate the application of these dressings and ensure the parents know what to do.

Less Common Abnormalities

Less commonly there are gross abnormalities, even to the extent of absence of the pinna and external auditory meatus. These are associated with deafness and middle ear abnormalities (Treacher–Collins, etc. see Chapter 12). In some of these children it may be possible to improve the hearing or at least to provide a pit for the acceptance of a hearing aid, though this would not generally be

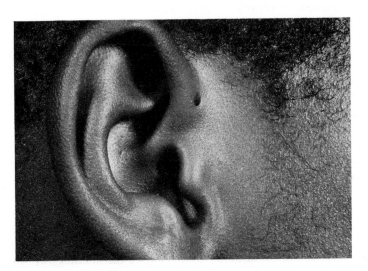

Fig. 6.1   Preauricular sinus. The opening of the sinus is seen as a tiny pit above the tragus and just in front of the helix; this is the typical site.

advised if the opposite ear were normal. Construction of a new pinna is a difficult procedure, generally undertaken by a plastic surgeon, and a compromise with the construction of an ear lobe, the remainder of the defect being hidden under the hair, or the use of a prosthesis may be more appropriate.

Other congenital abnormalities include the occurrence of *accessory auricles*, generally represented by firm small lumps of cartilage covered by skin below and in front of the pinna, and a *pre-auricular sinus* (Fig. 6.1) which is seen in front of the tragus as a blind pit (where there may be an underlying cyst) and a track leading down towards the tympanic membrane. These minor deformities may be ignored by the patient, otherwise they should be excised, particularly if a pre-auricular cyst discharges or the sinus becomes infected.

Infection

Perichondritis of the Pinna

This is an unusual condition, but of importance because it is likely to result in destruction and absorption of the cartilage and hence gross deformity of the ear. It is due to either a pyogenic infection of the perichondrium or to a progressive systemic condition in which elastic cartilage elsewhere in the body is affected (relapsing polychondritis).

Trauma

Wounds of the pinna bleed profusely and heal readily. Haematoma results from shearing of the skin and perichondrium over the underlying cartilage; traditionally held to be a boxing injury, it probably more commonly follows a rugby scrummage. There is no generally accepted correct way of treating this, as whether it is left, drained or aspirated, there is deformity and thickening of the pinna known as cauliflower ear.

EXTERNAL AUDITORY CANAL

Foreign Body

Not uncommonly, children put foreign bodies into their various orifices. Objects found in the ear include plastic beads, peas and nuts. The child may present with deafness if the foreign body is inert, or with an infected painful ear. Mother may have seen the child put something in the ear or may see it when the child is being washed. Rarely, insects get into the ear and the resulting noise and irritation can make the patient's behaviour bizarre. Foreign bodies may be removed in the outpatient department if the patient will keep still, but if he is reluctant or if there is much pain or oedema, it will have to be removed under general anaesthesia.

Otitis Externa

This common important condition of the external ear involves inflammation of the skin lining the cartilaginous part of the ear canal. Deafness and watery or purulent discharge may be present, but the dominating feature is generally pain which may keep the patient awake. Movement of the pinna is painful. The walls of the canal may be apposed by oedema closing the meatus. More deeply there is a collection of debris harbouring the responsible organisms. Local lymphadenitis, generally pre-auricular over the parotid gland but sometimes postauricular over the mastoid, if present, indicates the spread of infection. Otitis externa due to fungal infection may present as a pultaceous mass of mycelial debris and discharge, or in a dry ear (often with a quiescent CSOM or a dry mastoid cavity) when the hyphae can be seen under the microscope. Infection of a hair follicle presenting as a furuncle at the meatus is self limiting with resolution after the boil has been discharged, but a simple glycerine and ichthammol wick carefully inserted is comforting. In all other cases, the essential treatment is to clean the canal as thoroughly as possible, preferably with suction under a microscope. This is painful and needs extreme care but if trauma is avoided, the condition will resolve more quickly the cleaner the canal.

Suction Clearance

Suction clearance under the microscope is seldom performed by a nurse. However, this is one area into which the role of the nurse could usefully be extended. Obviously before undertaking this treatment a nurse needs time to observe and then practise under supervision. This can be facilitated by making use of the teaching arm extension of the microscope.

Before commencing suction clearance the canal is sometimes filled with normal saline or a bland detergent e.g. savlon. Gentle suction is then applied until the fluid is removed and the canal is clean.

After cleaning, drops containing steroid and antiseptic or antibiotic will be effective and if careful daily toilet at the outpatient department is possible, the patient is generally much better (and grateful) in 48 hours. The insertion of a dry compressed fibre wick which expands gently on adding the appropriate drops is recommended in the difficult acute case. The condition is prone to recur and search must then be made for an underlying cause, for example eczema or psoriasis of the canal. Some cases are associated with seborrhoea capitis. If the patient is in the habit of using hair dye or lacquer, the effect of a trial period without these should be observed. The continued ineffective use of a variety of drugs may induce sensitivity of the skin, causing further problems.

The patient must be told not to attempt to clean the ear blindly by poking it; in particular cotton wool buds should not be used, and this message driven home by a simple explanation of nature's way of cleaning it (see Chapter 2).

Malignant Otitis Externa

This rare but important condition in which infection spreads through the temporal bone, if left untreated, kills the patient after a period of intense pain. Diabetes is usually a feature and once diagnosed extensive surgical excision plus intensive antibiotic therapy, including metroanidazole, is the treatment of choice.

Osteomata

Osteomata of the external canal are bony irregularities of characteristic appearance. They form in those who have been swimming habitually in cold water in childhood and adolescence. Generally of no concern, being found in a symptomless ear, they will obscure the tympanic membrane to a variable extent and may prevent adequate toilet of the canal. With care they can simply be removed with a burr.

Aural Toilet

The aim of aural toilet is to remove discharge or debris present in the external auditory canal.

This is a surgically clean rather than a sterile procedure. Small loosely separated tufts of the finest quality cotton wool are firmly applied to a wool carrier, and this cannot be properly done using a non-touch technique. The most commonly used instrument is the wool carrier end of a Jobson Horne probe.

The best light source is a head mirror and Bull's eye lamp, as this then leaves both hands free for the dressing whilst maintaining constant direct vision of the canal.

The patient should be seated comfortably with his clothing protected. After examination, the ear is gently cleaned of all debris and discharge using circular movements of the wool carrier. The cotton wool is changed after each cleansing action.

When the canal has been cleaned as far as possible the prescribed drops or dressing are inserted. Medication can be applied to a wick, which is a piece of 1.25 cm ribbon gauze 10–13 cm long. The wick is inserted using Keen's or Tilley's aural dressing forceps. The patient should be told if the medication (e.g. glycerine and ichthammol) can stain fabric.

A small piece of cotton wool may be inserted at the entrance of the canal to absorb any discharge or medication.

Instillation of Ear Drops

Each patient must have his own bottle of ear drops, it should not be shared.

After explaining the procedure the nurse helps the patient into a comfortable lateral position. The affected ear is uppermost, one pillow under the head and the clothing protected.

The canal is straightened by gentle traction on the pinna and the drops instilled. After releasing the pinna, gentle pressing actions on the tragus may be used to 'pump' the drops down the canal. The patient should remain in the lateral position for 10 minutes before rising or having the procedure repeated to the other ear. A small piece of cotton wool can be inserted at the entrance of the canal as on the completion of aural toilet.

Wax

The normal healthy ear contains a certain amount of brown 'wax'. The material consists of the secretion of the ceruminous glands together with desquamated epithelial cells shed from the skin lining the canal and a variable amount of hair. Normally this migrates naturally to the external meatus but this movement is hindered if the hairs of the canal are tough (as in the elderly male) or if, as more commonly happens now, the patient, thinking he is cleaning the ears, pokes a cotton wool bud down the canal. Clearly this simply has the effect of pushing the material in the wrong direction.

Not infrequently wax becomes impacted in the canal and in time becomes very hard. It can be removed under direct vision or by syringing. If it is not readily dislodged by these means it can be softened by drops, for example of warm olive oil, given over a few days before a further attempt is made.

Ear Syringing

Ear syringing is carried out to remove excessive wax, foreign bodies or discharge from the ear canal.

The procedure should only be performed upon written instructions from a doctor, who should inspect the ear before and after the procedure.

A Wood's metal syringe (Fig. 6.2) which holds 120 ml of fluid is comfortable to hold and use. Other types of syringes available are the Bacon (Fig. 6.2) and Higginson rubber syringes. Large departments may have a tank with the pressure and temperature

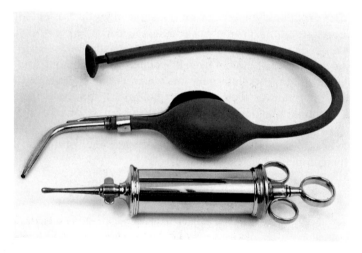

Fig. 6.2   Bacon's rubber ear syringe; Wood's metal ear syringe.

of the fluid automatically controlled. All equipment must run smoothly to maintain a steady even flow of fluid. Nozzles must always be attached firmly to prevent accidental dislodgement as this can damage the drum or canal. Fluids used include tap water, normal saline or a sodium bicarbonate solution.

After giving an explanation of the procedure, confirm that the patient has no knowledge of a dry perforation. If the likelihood of a perforation exists syringing should not be performed—wax etc. would then be removed under the microscope by a doctor. Syringing is not without possible hazards. The patient should be asked to indicate if he experiences any untoward symptoms, such as pain, vertigo or fluid running into the back of the throat. Should these occur syringing should stop.

The patient should sit comfortably with his clothing protected by a mackintosh and an absorbent towel.

The nurse examines the ear under direct vision to see the nature, size and position of what is to be removed. The temperature of the

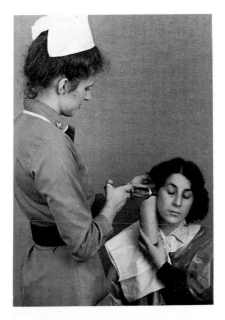

Fig. 6.3 Ear syringing. Note the position of the nurse. One hand is used to hold the pinna and straighten the canal while the syringe is held in the other hand. The patient is holding an aluminium receiver which is used to collect the return fluid during ear syringing.

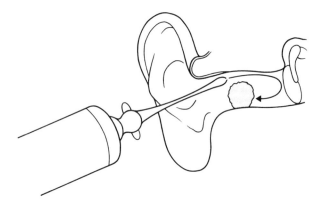

Fig. 6.4 Fluid is directed towards the posterior wall of the canal, and is seen passing behind wax or a foreign body.

solution is checked. It must be 38°C; if it is cooler, vertigo is a real possibility. The patient is asked to hold a receiver under his ear to collect the return fluid (Fig. 6.2). The syringe is filled and, pointing it upwards, air is expelled. The nurse stands to the side and slightly in front of the patient (Fig. 6.3). The canal is straightened by gentle traction on the pinna and the tip of the nozzle is inserted just inside the canal; it should always be in view. The fluid is directed in a steady even flow towards the posterior wall of the canal (Fig. 6.4). A guide to the target area is to compare the perimeter of the canal to a clock face—for the left ear direct the fluid towards 1 o'clock, for the right ear, 11 o'clock (Fig. 6.5).

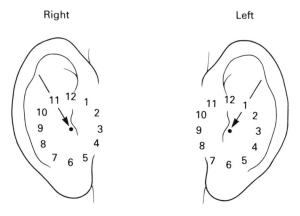

Fig. 6.5 The stream of fluid is directed towards the area indicated by the arrow.

Syringing is continued until the canal is clean. This is confirmed by further examination. The procedure should be completed within 10 minutes, otherwise syringing is stopped and the patient referred back to the doctor.

On completion, residual fluid in the canal can be drained by the patient tilting his head. The canal should then be gently mopped dry using cotton wool on a wool carrier.

7 Secretory Otitis Media (Glue Ear)

The commonest cause of deafness in Caucasian children is fluid filling the middle ear—in other races the incidence is uncertain, but may well be less. Often the fluid is tenacious and resists easy aspiration by suction, hence the term 'glue ear'. Possibly more than 20% of children are affected at some time and screening for deafness in schools is now common. Nowadays the commonest operation in Britain is for glue ear, whereas previously the commonest procedure was adenotonsillectomy. Untreated this condition eventually resolves spontaneously and rarely persists into adult life. However, the hearing is impaired while the glue remains; in some cases there is deterioration in the quality of the tympanic membrane, which becomes indrawn, and in time a retraction pocket with formation of cholesteatoma may result.

AETIOLOGY

The aetiology is unknown. Normally the tiny amounts of mucus secreted in the middle ear escape into the nasopharynx via the Eustachian tube, and the middle ear remains aerated. Whether the failure of 'glue' to drain is due to its physical properties or whether on the other hand the Eustachian tube is initially at fault so that the middle ear is inadequately aerated and fluid accumulates, is not clear. In the past it has been suggested that hypertrophy of the adenoids and of adjacent lymphoid tissue effectively blocks the Eustachian tube orifice and this has been the rationale for adenoidectomy as part of the treatment. If there is nasal obstruction from the adenoid mass then adenoidectomy is indicated—but otherwise it is without proven effect in the management of glue ear. Other suggestions have included immunological deficiencies,

allergies, and that it is the result of acute infection that has been
only partially treated by antibiotics.

PRESENTATION

The condition presents as a hearing loss. This becomes apparent
initially either to the parent or teacher, but all too often before the
deafness is recognized, the child has been considered to be naughty
or disobedient. Typical features of the history are that the child
does not hear when called from another room, and likes the radio
or television turned up. Pain in the ear is not usually a symptom
and when it occurs it is not severe or prolonged.

EXAMINATION

The child's deafness to the whispered voice in the consulting room
is not always obvious. In most cases the appearance of the
tympanic membrane is characteristic—it may be hyperaemic, dull
grey, or have an orange tinge, but whatever its colour it tends to
lose its normal translucence and become retracted. Use of the
Siegle speculum reveals impairment of movement of the tympanic
membrane. Tuning fork tests show a conductive hearing loss. Due
to the incompressibility of the fluid, the impedance tympanograms
show a flat curve, that is, changing the pressure does not affect the
position or shape of the tympanic membrane. The presence of fluid
causes a hearing loss of 30 dB over the low frequencies. However,
the young child may have normal hearing of better than 0 dB (say
-5 or -10) so that the pure tone threshold may be 20 dB in the
presence of glue.

MANAGEMENT

Medical Treatment

Medical treatment to date is aimed at improving Eustachian tube
function by topical vasoconstricting nasal sprays or drops (see
Chapter 18 for procedure) and by antihistamines or similar drugs
which have the effect of shrinking the nasal mucosa. Alternatively,

treatment is aimed at liquifying the tenacious mucus in the hope that it can escape. Neither treatment is of proven benefit. If the middle ear can be inflated with Politzerisation (see Fig. 3.6), there is a good rationale for having the child, if sufficiently co-operative, blow up an inflatable toy using the nose; this should be repeated several times a day. When this is successful in inflating the ears, the child by a gesture will often indicate something has happened in the ear. The hearing is immediately better but the improvement only lasts whilst the air is still present.

Surgical Treatment

Surgical treatment is aimed at aerating the middle ear. Except in those few cases where the fluid is thin, it cannot be completely aspirated via a myringotomy. In these circumstances, most surgeons would insert a grommet into the tympanic membrane (Fig. 7.1). Provided this stays in position and does not become blocked either with blood or secretions, it ensures that the middle ear contains air and one expects hearing improvement to be apparent as soon as the child recovers from the anaesthetic.

Some surgeons advise against swimming and stipulate that the ear is occluded with cotton wool smeared with Vaseline when the hair is washed because of the danger of water entering the middle

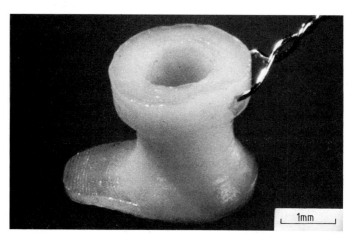

Fig. 7.1   A grommet, provided with a wire to aid removal. However, commonly it is used without this wire.

ear and causing infection. However, experiments show that, because of the small size of the hole in the grommet, and surface tension, water will not go through the grommet unless it is under pressure. In the public swimming bath water the content of viable bacteria is strictly controlled. But the disinfectant may irritate the lining of the upper air passages inducing a 'chemical rhinitis' which then becomes secondarily infected producing sinusitis or otitis media. (These events may occur whether the child has a grommet or not.) Even if the middle ear becomes infected and there is a purulent discharge through the grommet, generally no great harm is done. These risks should be weighed against the importance of swimming to the child, and most otologists would not advise against swimming for children with grommets provided they do not dive or swim underwater.

Often the grommet will be extruded spontaneously within 12 months and further management depends on the findings when the child is reviewed. If glue has reaccumulated bilaterally, insertion of a further grommet or grommets would be advised. The problem tends to recur and many (about 30%) of the children who have a grommet inserted will eventually have at least one further one. With repeated insertion of grommets there is scarring of the tympanic membrane. On the other hand, if the condition is untreated or inadequately treated, there is often deterioration of the tympanic membrane, as previously described. If at any time there is a discharge of pus through the grommet from an infection of the middle ear it is probably advisable to leave the tube *in situ* and treat with an antibiotic. Although generally infections will not resolve in the presence of a foreign body, this does not necessarily apply in the case of a grommet.

Usually the condition affects both ears—if only one is affected and the hearing is good in the unaffected ear, interference is not necessarily indicated as the child with one good-hearing ear is not sufficiently handicapped. However, follow-up is needed because if on the affected side the quality of the TM begins to deteriorate (thinning or becoming further retracted) the insertion of a grommet may well reverse this process.

When conservative management is preferred or when repeated grommet insertion fails to inflate the middle ear (e.g. because the grommets become blocked or extruded early) the provision of a hearing aid should be considered.

As an alternative to a grommet, a Goode's T tube may be used

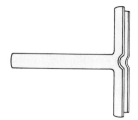

Fig. 7.2   A Goode's T-tube.

(Fig. 7.2). This has a larger lumen and because of the length of the flanges, it is not so readily extruded and may be expected to maintain aeration of the middle ear for a longer period than a grommet. It is perhaps of particular value in those cases in which grommet insertion has failed to control the disease (e.g. because the grommet has become blocked or extruded prematurely) or when the quality of the tympanic membrane has deteriorated significantly.

Glue ear is a common problem but difficult to explain to parents and it is recommended therefore, that they be given a simple explanatory leaflet, particularly if surgical treatment is recommended.

NURSING CARE FOR MYRINGOTOMY AND INSERTION OF GROMMET

Pre-operative Objectives

1   To give the family adequate information about the ward and pre- and postoperative events.
2   To provide emotional and psychological support for the family.
3   To prepare the child physically and emotionally for a general anaesthetic.
4   To ensure good communication and relations between the staff and the family, taking into account the child's hearing loss.

Pre-operative Care

Almost all that is written on the care of a child prior to tonsillectomy also applies here (refer to Chapter 25 for details). The care has not been duplicated but important points stressed and additional features included. Again this is very possibly the child's first hospital admission and preparation for this experience should start in the outpatient area when the decision to operate is taken. As well as the parents, the child should be given suitable explanations at this stage.

In most cases the child is admitted the day before the operation, but if adenoidectomy is not scheduled, admission as a day case is feasible. The importance of including the parents in the care of their child whilst he is in hospital is now more fully appreciated. Play is a very important part of a child's day and is essential, whether in or out of hospital, for well being.

A paediatric nursing history sheet or questionnaire is used on admission to gain information about the child, from the child himself and his parents. Vital signs will need to be recorded and a ward urinalysis performed. Drug dosage is calculated according to weight, making accurate assessment of the child's weight essential. If a haemoglobin estimation is required blood should be taken. The surgeon may request that audiometry testing is repeated; this usually depends on how much time has elapsed since the last audiogram.

In order to gain the child's trust simple explanations are given about the reasons for the various investigations. The need to starve prior to general anaesthesia is also explained. Some children may also have a sensorineural hearing loss (see p. 100). There are many possible reasons for this and such children will be wearing hearing aids, and may lip read (see p. 104). Without the hearing aids the child may have virtually no hearing so it is important that the aids are in good working order and are removed only when anaesthesia has been induced. Important points related to communication with any person who lip-reads are described in Chapter 11.

Post-operative Care

Following complete recovery from anaesthesia the child can be nursed in bed in the position that he finds most comfortable. When the child is able, fluids can be given, followed by a more solid diet as condition and appetite dictate. The time that the child is under general anaesthesia is usually quite short, and many children will be wide awake, bored and hungry within 6 hours. At this stage the presence of mother to read or to play gently is invaluable both for the child and the nursing staff.

Children who are well enough can be carried or escorted to the bathroom for toilet purposes later in the day, and they may comment that a common event such as flushing the toilet is much noisier. Many children find potties just as undignified and difficult to use as adults find bed pans.

There may be a little serous blood-stained discharge from the ear on the day of operation, which can be gently wiped away from the entrance to the canal with sterile cottonwool dressed applicators.

As soon as the child is able to tolerate it, any hearing aid should be reinserted. The ear piece should be cleaned and dried before insertion.

After Care

When the child is ready to go home it is important that the parents appreciate the major part they have to play in the continuing care. Advice needs to be given and opportunities for questions made available; it is often better if verbal instructions are reinforced with written instructions as these can be kept for future reference.

The child can return to school when the parents consider him fit, usually within 1 week of discharge. If a grommet has been inserted a plug of cotton wool smeared with Vaseline, or an ear plug may be used when washing the hair or bathing (see p. 60). This applies for as long as a grommet is *in situ* and for 1 week following myringotomy provided there have been no complications.

It is important that follow-up appointments are kept even if the child's hearing appears normal and he has been free of ear problems. This often needs to be stressed.

When a grommet has been inserted it is necessary to explain what it does (it is there to allow air into the middle ear, rather than to drain fluid) and that it is likely to come out of its own accord within the next year or so. As one of the parents is the most likely person to find the grommet after it has been extruded, it is wise to show them one (Fig. 7.1). It is possible that the child may complain of a sensation of fullness, popping or clicking in the ear and this is not harmful. If once the child goes home there is bleeding, discharge or pain, he should be seen by the GP.

8 Other Conditions of the Middle Ear

INFECTIVE

Acute Suppurative Otitis Media

ASOM is a common condition in childhood. During the first year of schooling it will occur at least once in 20% of children in Britain. This high incidence is undoubtedly related to the frequency of upper respiratory tract infections (URTI) at this age. These produce inflammation of the nasal and pharyngeal mucosa; the Eustachian tube is also involved and becomes blocked. Such a closed off cavity readily becomes infected, although another possibility is that infected nasal secretions may gain access via the Eustachian tube while it is patent, particularly if driven in by nose blowing. The commonest infecting organisms are *Staphylococcus pyogenes* (40%), *Streptococcus haemolyticus* (30%) and *S. pneumococcus* (10%). With the increasing production of pus under tension, there is thrombosis of the vulnerable vessels in the unsupported tympanic membrane which eventually leads, if the infection is not arrested, to perforation of the tympanic membrane and a discharge of the pus.

ASOM in the adult is uncommon. When it occurs it often follows URTI or barotrauma, but it is important to search for other causes of obstruction to the Eustachian tube (e.g. a tumour) by examination of the nose and post nasal space (PNS).

Clinical Features

The typical history in the child is of rapidly increasing pain in the ear, following a 'cold'. Commonly this will waken the child at night and the parents feel helpless and anxious. When the tympanic membrane perforates, which may happen within a few hours, there is a release of pus and relief of pain. In almost all cases the discharge will cease within a few days and the perforation will heal, though the hearing may take a few weeks to return to normal. Acute otitis media occasionally affects the baby, producing fever and restlessness, and there may be features of gastro-enteritis, but the diagnosis may not be obvious until otorrhoea is found. It is also a complication of measles and whooping cough. The ears of children with these infections should be examined.

On the other hand, otalgia is a common symptom—perhaps the commonest symptom leading to a medical consultation—and particularly common in children. In the vast majority of such cases the pain resolves without any undue sequelae. Unless there is otoscopic evidence these should not be labelled as infections and an analgesic is more appropriate than a course of antibiotic.

Treatment

If a systemic antibiotic, e.g. amoxicillin, is given in time, the pain is eased and the tympanic membrane will not rupture. Nevertheless, the effusion in the middle ear may persist for a variable period and the hearing may not recover for several weeks. In the early recovery phase the tympanic membrane has a characteristic appearance with white stripes of desquamating epithelium radiating from its centre.

Complications (Fig. 8.1)

MASTOIDITIS

The infection in the middle ear cavity may extend into the adjacent mastoid air cells. If this results in tenderness over the mastoid the diagnosis of 'mastoiditis' is made. There may be oedema and hyperaemia of the skin immediately behind the ear in the post-auricular groove, with displacement of the pinna outwards and forwards. Mastoiditis may occur together with a purulent otorrhoea, but perhaps more commonly nowadays it is found in children who have acute otitis media without rupture of the tympanic membrane. Generally such children will have had a course of antibiotics for a few days with relief of the acute otalgia, and the diagnosis may thus be delayed.

Treatment in hospital with an intensive course of parenteral antibiotics generally cures the condition. The child should be kept

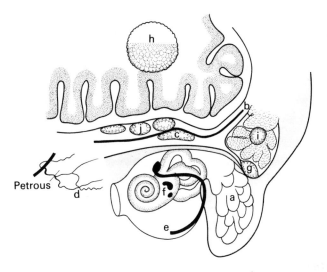

Fig. 8.1 The complications of middle ear infection. (a) Mastoiditis; (b) meningitis; (c) extradural abscess; (d) petrositis; (e) facial nerve paralysis; (f) labyrinthitis; (g) lateral sinus thrombosis; (h) temporal lobe abscess; (i) cerebellar abscess; (j) subdural abscess. (Adapted by kind permission from Foxen E. H. M. (1980) *Lecture Notes on Diseases of the Ear, Nose and Throat*, 5th edn., p. 46. Blackwell Scientific Publications, Oxford.)

in bed until any pyrexia subsides. An analgesic will be required for the relief of pain and some, for example paracetamol, are doubly useful as they have an antipyretic effect. Vital signs are recorded at intervals determined by the child's condition. If there is otorrhoea aural toilet will be necessary (see Chapter 5). The canal and pinna need to be kept free of discharge which, if left to collect and dry, can cause otitis externa. The diet should be fluid, as long as a sufficient volume is given, until the child feels able to tolerate solids.

Surgery (cortical mastoidectomy) will be needed if the condition fails to resolve or if breakdown of bony trabeculae leads to abscess formation. Such an abscess may present over the mastoid bone, in the neck, in the posterior meatal wall or even in front of the ear.

SIGMOID SINUS THROMBOSIS

With the spread of infection through the bone there is a danger of its reaching the sigmoid sinus leading to thrombosis and infective thrombophlebitis. This is a life threatening condition. Retrograde spread of the thrombosis may impair the reabsorption of CSF, which will therefore accumulate producing otitic hydrocephalus.

Treatment is by an injection of intramuscular penicillin followed by a 7 day course of oral penicillin or ampicillin, unless the patient is known to be allergic to penicillin, in which case erythromycin is probably next best. If the tympanic membrane has not ruptured some surgeons advocate myringotomy to release the pus and relieve pain; this also allows a swab to be taken for culture and sensitivity. When possible, a head mirror and bullseye lamp are used while taking an ear swab. If the canal is to be straightened and a speculum inserted this is done very gently as the area is likely to be tender. The swab is passed through the speculum into the canal and rotated to collect as much cell debris and pus as possible.

CHRONIC SUPPURATIVE OTITIS MEDIA (CSOM)
Following ASOM, discharge will persist or be intermittent if the function of the Eustachian tube does not recover. Possible underlying causes for this include sinusitis and persistent mouth breathing—malnutrition from hypovitaminosis is an important feature in patients with CSOM in many countries.

If healing does not take place within a few weeks the condition of CSOM develops in which there is a perforation and through this can be seen red oedematous mucosa on the medial wall of the middle ear. The presence of the perforation itself predisposes to further attacks of acute infection, which may reach the middle ear either from the external canal or from the pharynx, as infected material is more likely to be blown into such an ear via the Eustachian tube than when the middle ear is a closed cavity.

The amount and character of the discharge varies, at times being mucoid when there is no bacterial infection, at times frankly purulent or muco purulent, and these alternate with dry periods. The perforation is generally anteroinferior; the posterosuperior part is not involved except as part of a large perforation, in which case the malleus is pulled inwards by the tensor tympani muscle and may rest on the promontory, appearing simply as a stump. In such a florid case there may well be necrosis of the long process of the incus and hence 'ossicular discontinuity'. A localized exuberant area of inflamed mucosa may progress through a stage of 'granulation' to form an aural polyp which appears as a red lump in the external auditory canal.

NON-INFECTIVE

'CSOM' with Cholesteatoma

This form of middle ear disease is also referred to as CSOM in books but this term can be criticized as in this disease, unlike the one just described, infection probably takes no part in the aetiology and it by no means always occurs in the established condition, and a discharge of pus is not a universal feature. It is increasingly considered nowadays that cholesteatoma (apart from the rare congenital cholesteatoma) results from retraction of the tympanic membrane as a result of poor Eustachian tube function (see Chapter 7). It is probably significant that this retraction is most pronounced in the regions furthest away from the Eustachian tube orifice, that is, in the attic and the aditus. As the process extends, these areas become cut off from the rest of the middle ear cavity, and from the Eustachian tube. A pocket is then formed, the lining of which is continuous with the external layer of the tympanic membrane. This continues to desquamate. Provided the shed epithelium can escape, through the self-cleansing pocket, no great harm is done, but if the sac becomes sufficiently deep, the squames cannot escape and the collection of epithelial debris is called cholesteatoma. This sac has the ability to slowly expand, destroying bone as it enlarges. Precisely how this happens is not agreed at present. Some authorities believe that cholesteatma may arise from middle ear mucosa which has changed to a squamous epithelium termed squamous metaplasia.

Clinical Features

There is a foul smelling discharge and deafness. On examination, it may be possible to see the cholesteatoma sac or the white debris of its shed epithelium. The mouth of the sac may be seen, either superiorly (in the attic region) or posterosuperiorly.

Management

Management depends very much on the age and general condition of the patient. One sees patients who give a history of intermittent trouble with the ear for over 50 years and the cholesteatoma is posing little threat, but in general, mastoidectomy would be recommended if the patient is otherwise fit.

MASTOIDECTOMY

The primary objective of this operation is to eradicate disease. In cortical mastoidectomy for mastoiditis, the bone is drilled out and unhealthy mucosa removed; the middle ear structures are left *in situ*. When dealing with cholesteatoma, the further aim is to fashion a smooth mastoid cavity, without pockets, so that there is no possibility of squamous epithelium re-accumulating. Generally this can only be accomplished by removing at least some of the middle ear ossicles (however, these are often at least partially destroyed by disease).

Tympanoplasty

After the disease has been removed, attempts to reconstruct the hearing mechanism may, in some cases, be worthwhile. Some surgeons would do this at a second operation having allowed the ear to settle down and new healthy epithelium to grow. The tympanic membrane can be reconstructed (myringoplasty) using a connective tissue graft and the ossicular chain reconstructed (ossiculoplasty) using either a bone graft or synthetic materials. If both myringoplasty and ossiculoplasty are performed the procedure may be termed a tympanoplasty.

Complications (Fig. 8.1)

It is considered a potentially dangerous condition, because with insidious extension it can lead to sigmoid sinus thrombosis, meningitis, and brain abscesses of either the temporal lobe superiorly via the floor of the middle cranial fossa or alternatively of the cerebellum posteriorly.

TRAUMA

Head injury may produce a fracture of the temporal bone and if this involves the middle ear it can cause ossicular disruption, haemorrhagic effusion in the middle ear or a tear of the tympanic membrane or of the meatal wall with bleeding from the ear. A slap on the ear can tear the tympanic membrane. A perforation or haemorrhagic middle ear effusion may also result from an increase in ambient pressure (otic barotrauma) on descent when diving or in an aircraft if the pressure has not been equalized via the Eustachian tube.

These tears of the tympanic membrane heal spontaneously within a few weeks and effusions will absorb. It is often possible to reconnect the ossicular chain if this has been disrupted.

OTOSCLEROSIS

In this condition there is active bone growth of the stapes footplate and the adjacent area of the oval window. This produces 'stapes fixation' and hence a conductive hearing loss. With progress of the disease there is also sensorineural hearing loss attributed to cochlear involvement which may also be an early feature. In the 1950s many of these patients were treated by fenestration in which effectively a new 'oval window' was drilled in the side of the lateral semicircular canal via a mastoidectomy approach. Some of these patients are still seen in ENT clinics for cleansing of their mastoid cavities. In the 1960s stapedectomy became popular and gave good results, but some patients were left with a 'dead ear', which may occur after an initially good result, while other patients may have a distressing tinnitus. There is increasingly a more conservative approach in British practice therefore, and a hearing aid is often recommended if this is feasible and acceptable.

Rarely, congenitally fixed, absent or misshapen middle ear ossicles occur, and produce a conductive hearing loss from birth.

CARE PRIOR TO EAR SURGERY

Most patients will have known the date and time of their admission for days or weeks in advance. The nursing staff also have this information and it is possible to make preparations so that the patient feels expected and welcome on arrival. A warm, friendly welcome and introduction to some of the staff and other patients can help reduce anxiety. Objectives for pre-operative care are outlined in Chapter 1.

Effective Communication

The nursing history or questionnaire should be completed in a quiet, well lit area to aid communication between the nurse, patient and any other person who may be present. It is essential to establish good communication with the patient before surgery, particularly if hearing may be reduced postoperatively by bandages, and any means the patient uses to supplement hearing, for example lip reading, must be noted in the nursing records.

Patients with a BE hearing aid should be informed if a loop system has been installed in the ward sitting/television room as their aid may have a pick-up coil which can be used to listen to radio or television. Alternatively another type of environmental aid may be offered.

Infection

It is wise to establish whether there is any otorrhoea (which would indicate inflammation or infection) from the ear which is to be operated on, before admitting the patient. Some operations, for example myringoplasty, may not be performed if there is otorrhoea. If there is any doubt about whether or not the operation will be performed medical advice should be sought before continuing with admission. Being admitted into hospital and psychologically prepared for surgery unnecessarily is a traumatic experience. The patient will need to know why surgery is not possible at this time to avoid the incident being repeated. An OPD appointment, and probably medications to treat the problem, will be given before the patient is asked to return home.

Skin Preparation

Before removing any hair from the site of incision, the nurse must make sure that the patient has been seen and examined by a doctor and the consent form has been signed. Always check with the written records and with the patient whether the operation is to be performed on the right or left ear (sometimes both ears are affected by disease). The type of incision or approach will determine the area which requires hair removal. If in doubt, check. Unnecessary and extensive hair removal is a mistake that a patient has to live with for several weeks. The scalp and hair must be clean and free from lice and nits. The most convenient way to prepare the hair for removal is to make a parting using the patient's comb, along the outer edge of the area to be cleared of hair. Comb all hair above or to the side of this line away from the area. It may be necessary to hold this hair in position with hair grips, soft soap or a hair fixative; long hair can be tied away from the area with a piece of tape or ribbon gauze. The required area can then be cleared without adjacent hair getting in the way. Any long hairs present in the external auditory meatus will be cut in the operating theatre. At the end of the procedure the hair can be allowed to fall back into its normal style. Hair grips must not be used when the patient is going for operation, but long hair can be combed away from the prepared area and tied with tape or ribbon gauze before the premedication is given. An elastic band should not be used for this purpose as it is very uncomfortable.

Knowledge of Postoperative Events

The surgery is often planned for the day following admission which can mean that there is less than 24 hours for mental and physical preparation. During this time the patient will be seen by at least one member of the medical staff and possibly have several tests performed, for example, X-rays, audiogram, full blood count and electrocardiogram. When the preparation time is so short it is of vital importance that the nurse responsible for the patient's care ensures that there is time to discuss the pre-operative preparation and anticipated postoperative events thoroughly. Such events could include describing the method used to check the VII cranial nerve and the presence of a pressure bandage. If applicable, the instructions regarding nose blowing and sneezing (p. 81) should be described.

The patient's understanding of the aims of the surgery should be sought as not all operations on the ear are done to improve hearing. For example, the aims of the radical mastoidectomy operation is to make the ear and surrounding area safe from further complications of the disease, not to improve hearing.

If successful, surgery on the ear can greatly improve the quality of a person's life. Hearing may be dramatically improved so that social isolation and frustration are reduced, and water sports played and enjoyed once again. Neither of these may be possible, but if the problems associated with constant, or intermittent otorrhoea are removed, then this is an achievement. When so much is at stake the patient will be anxious before and after surgery until some indication of success or failure can be given. During this time a nurse must gain insight into, and understanding of the patient's fears and worries. A sympathetic but positive attitude shown when caring for this patient will help in building up a relationship based on confidence and trust.

CARE FOLLOWING EAR SURGERY

It is necessary to help the patient maintain a position which will minimize pain and enhance healing. Initially the most comfortable and suitable position is the lateral one with the operated ear uppermost. If the patient lies with the operated ear undermost he will invariably become uncomfortable and try to move about to relieve the pain and pressure. Restlessness can also stimulate vertigo, nausea and vomiting. After delicate operations on the middle ear the surgeon may give specific instructions regarding the position of the patient. When he is ready, the patient can be helped into a more comfortable position. Mobilization may begin on the day following operation.

Haemorrhage and Infection

Dressings and bandages should be observed for haemorrhage and to ensure that they are neither too slack nor too tight. The pressure dressing and bandage is applied following ear surgery to prevent bleeding and haematoma formation, so it needs to be quite firm. If the bandage has been applied so tightly that it is cutting into the soft tissues and causing severe discomfort or pain then it will need to be cut (over the forehead) but left in position and another bandage applied. It is wise to consult a doctor before pursuing this course of action. Sometimes the first bandage applied in theatre is too slack and another firmer bandage needs to be applied over the existing one. Should blood or serous fluid stains appear on the bandage, note the size, by marking the circumference with a pen or pencil, and the time it occurred for future comparison. It is impossible to state the right time for the inexperienced ENT nurse to inform a doctor when there is some oozing through the bandage. However, there will always be a senior nurse on duty who should be called for advice. If there are any doubts, or if the stain can be seen to be enlarging, it is definitely the right time, even for the experienced. In most instances a wad of sterile gauze or cotton wool will be placed over the existing bandage and another firm bandage applied. It is rare that the initial bandage needs to be removed or the patient returned to the operating theatre for the treatment of haemorrhage. In order to promote healing and prevent infection, dressing procedures require an aseptic technique. A pressure bandage is usually removed 24–48 hours after surgery. Removal of this large and firm dressing gives the patient much relief but may cause him to feel faint or giddy, so this

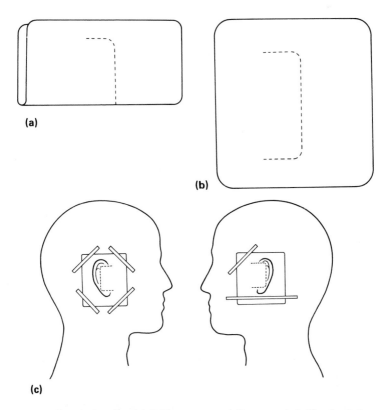

Fig. 8.2 An ear dressing. (a) Fold gauze or melolin square in half and cut shape outlined (the size of the cut is determined by the size of the patient); (b) this shape can be used for the right or left ear by simply turning the dressing over; (c) once in position the dressing is secured with strapping.

procedure is best done with the patient in bed. Following removal of the dressing it is necessary to inspect the wound for infection (as indicated by swelling, redness and undue tenderness), swelling due to haematoma formation, or discharge (from the wound or canal) and to check healing of the wound edges. If the wound is satisfactory then possibly only an aerosol plastic 'skin' dressing need be applied. A small gauze or Melolin dressing may be preferred in which case it should be changed daily (Fig. 8.2) until no longer required. If the patient wears spectacles the aerosol skin dressing should not be used alone as it will not afford the wound sufficient protection from the arm of the spectacles.

Drain Removal

Drains are rarely used except following acute mastoid surgery when they are left in place until drainage ceases (about 48 hours). Some surgeons do not suture the drain in position, which means that the drain will invariably come out when the pressure dressing is removed. It is wise to check the operation notes before starting such dressing so that the patient and the nurse know what to expect.

If there is a haematoma then this should be reported to the doctor concerned who will decide on treatment. This may involve removal of a suture and evacuation by gentle expression followed by the application of another dressing and bandage or alternatively, a small drain may be inserted.

Dressing Changes

If for any reason a patient requires frequent dressing changes then it is much kinder to apply a light bandage rather than strapping to hold the dressing in place; frequent changing of adhesive strapping which is attached to facial skin and hair is painful. A young child will need a light bandage to hold any dressing in place, and to protect the wound from his prying and often non-too-clean fingers. A method for applying an ear bandage is illustrated in Fig. 8.3. It is impossible to brush or comb the hair properly with an ear bandage on, so this needs to be done when the bandage is changed. Sutures may be continuous or interrupted, and remain in place for 5–7 days.

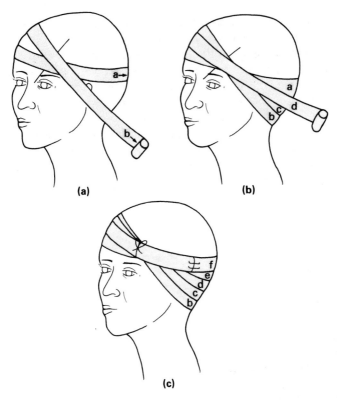

Fig. 8.3 Bandaging the ear. (a) Place ½ or 1 inch ribbon gauze tie on forehead, the bandage is usually 2–3 inches wide; (b) take first turn of bandage straight across the forehead and ear; (c) take second turn to bottom of ear dressing; (d) subsequent turns work up, and cover, the ear dressing; (e) secure end of bandage with strapping or a safety pin; (f) bring ends of ribbon gauze tie together and tie with a small bow; (g) check that the bandage is not too tight or too slack.

Ear Packs

Following most ear operations there will be a pack in the ear which remains in position for several weeks. A small piece of cotton wool is placed at the entrance of the canal to protect the pack and keep it clean. This piece of cotton wool should be changed as necessary.

VII Nerve Damage

Nursing responsibility for checking function of the VII cranial nerve normally commences in the recovery area of the operating theatre. The nurse who accepts the patient as being fit to return to the ward area should be told by, or ask, the recovery nurse about facial nerve function. In the ward area the VII nerve function is checked and recorded hourly at first then, if all is well, gradually reduced along with observations of vital signs. In order to check the nerve it is necessary to ask the patient to smile, wrinkle the nose, close the eyes tightly and raise the eyebrows. Damage to the nerve is shown by asymmetry of facial muscle movements. Even during recovery from anaesthesia asymmetric movement of the dilator nares may give early evidence of VII nerve damage. The facial muscles on the paralysed side do not move and the various skin creases which become apparent during muscle movement are also absent on this side. The upper eyelid on the paralysed side is unable to move down to cover the eyeball. (The muscle responsible for keeping the upper lid elevated is served by the III cranial nerve, and so its function is preserved.) Any asymmetry of muscle movement must be reported to the medical staff immediately, as it may be necessary to return the patient to the operating theatre for an exploratory operation in an attempt to identify and treat the cause of the paralysis. Pressure from a haematoma or a pack may be responsible for a facial palsy of delayed onset (see Chapter 9).

The chorda tympani, which is a branch of the VII nerve, may have been damaged or divided at the time of surgery. This nerve serves the ipsilateral anterior two-thirds of the tongue governing taste (sweet, sour and salt) so that a patient may complain of an alteration in taste. The most common complaint is that everything tastes rather bitter, as the taste buds which convey this sensation are on the posterior third of the tongue and these become dominant. Many patients will only give this information in passing as they put the alteration in taste down to hospital food! Taste will gradually return to normal.

Hypotension

Following ear surgery vital signs are recorded at intervals, according to the needs of the individual patient. If a hypotensive anaesthetic has been given, observation of pulse and blood pressure should be maintained until they have stabilized at the pre-operative level.

Nausea and Vomiting

Nausea and vomiting may be present in varying degrees following middle ear surgery, owing to the position of the sensitive vestibular apparatus. These are very distressing side-effects and if prolonged are likely to make even the most lively of personalities feel wretched and miserable. A sympathetic and caring attitude towards the patient can do much to relieve distress. An emesis bowl, tissues, mouth wash and receiver should always be on the patient's locker ready for use. Anti-emetics, for example prochlorperazine (Stemetil), are usually prescribed in anticipation of these problems and should be given when needed. Occasionally fluid loss from vomiting may be large enough to warrant a fluid balance chart.

The patient's food must be attractively presented and in a tolerable form, which may mean a fluid only diet. There are many preparations available that are palatable, contain the essential nutrients and sufficient calories, and can be given in liquid form, for example 'Build-up' or 'Clinifeed'. As nausea and vomiting subside a normal diet is gradually re-introduced. Provided there is no nausea or vomiting, fluids can be offered when the patient has sufficiently recovered from the anaesthetic.

Vertigo

Many patients experience vertigo and most find that it gradually diminishes as mobility increases. Explain to the patient that sudden movements of the head either to the side or forward can provoke vertigo. Vertigo can be kept to a minimum by moving the head slowly and by crouching down with the back straight to pick up something, rather than bending forward. One of the first movements that patients are likely to make when getting out of bed is to bend forward to find their slippers; it is important to warn against making this movement. The nurse should always be prepared to help patients put on their slippers, irrespective of how well they may appear. When vertigo is otherwise troublesome mobilization will need to be slower than normal and many patients find Cooksey-Cawthorne exercises helpful. These involve patients going through a variety of movements and changes of position, initially under supervision from the physiotherapist, so that they gradually regain confidence.

When patients are mobile they can bathe in the bathroom rather than in bed. Initially a nurse should help the patient in and out of the bath in case vertigo occurs. Showers can be taken if the operated ear and the suture line are completely covered by a waterproof shower cap.

Pain

The amount of pain experienced will vary according to the individual and the extent of the surgery. Removal of any pressure dressing frequently reduces pain and discomfort.

Hearing Loss

Although in some instances the operation will improve hearing, this may not be apparent whilst the patient is in hospital especially when there is packing in the ear. Communication between the patients and those caring for them must be a two-way process and Chapter 11 describes ways in which good communication can be maintained. It is important that the patient is able to take part in activities available in the ward, such as watching television or listening to the radio. Headphones with a louder than average volume range are available.

Discharge Advice

Before discharge, adequate information about convalescence must be given to the patient. Many patients are now discharged before sutures are removed so the period spent at home before returning to normal daily living patterns is lengthened. When the list of 'do's' and 'dont's' is lengthy it is always wise to consider giving written information which can be used for future reference by the patient and any other person involved. Written information never replaces verbal explanation; it merely supplements it and acts as a record.

The following information should be given to the patient before discharge.
1   The place, date and time for removal of sutures and packing.
2   The name, frequency and dosage of any medication to be continued at home should be clearly marked on the container provided by Pharmacy, and the reason for the medication should be clearly explained.

3 The hair can be washed once sutures have been removed. A piece of cotton wool smeared with vaseline, or an ear plug should be used during hair washing and bathing to prevent water entering the canal. Advise the patient to ask the doctor in OPD when this practice can be discontinued.

4 Any pack in the ear should be protected with a small piece of cotton wool placed at the entrance to the canal. This will need to be changed as necessary. The patient should be shown how to change the cotton wool and be given some cotton wool balls. Stress that the hands should be thoroughly washed and dried before touching the piece of cotton wool which is to be inserted. There may be a small amount of discharge coming through the pack. This is acceptable, but if the discharge becomes offensive, copious, purulent or blood stained the patient should return to the hospital.

5 Following reconstructive middle ear surgery the patient should initially avoid situations where there is likely to be a change in atmospheric pressure, for example an aeroplane or underground train, as this can affect the position of any graft or prosthesis. The doctor will tell the patient when it is considered safe to be in such a situation be it for work or pleasure. Violent nose blowing and sneezing can also alter middle ear pressure and should be discouraged. The nose can be blown gently one side at a time. It is impossible to sneeze gently, but attempts can be made to stifle a sneeze, or if this also proves impossible the patient should try to sneeze with his mouth open.

6 All water sports are contraindicated until medical approval is given.

7 The length of time that absence from work or school is recommended will vary according to the individual; advice from the general practitioner or OPD doctor should be sought.

8 In order to reduce the likelihood of an upper respiratory tract infection, which may spread to the middle ear, places where there are large groups of people or any person who has such an infection should be avoided if at all possible.

9 An OPD appointment will be given.

10 Patients should be aware of whether it is considered acceptable practice for them to telephone the ward or OPD with any queries or problems they might have, or whether they are expected to seek advice from their general practitioner who will be notified about the surgery and any subsequent care required.

11 If there is any vertigo at all then the patient must not drive.

Much of this information will be given by a doctor, but the nurse should still ensure that the patient has received and understood it. In some instances it may prove necessary for a member of the Community Nursing Services to take over care until such time as the patient is completely fit. It is particularly important to inform these services about the discharge of any patient who had been receiving their care before admission into hospital.

9   Conditions of the Inner Ear

CONGENITAL

Malformations of the inner ear present as deafness from birth. In about 50% of cases there is either a relevant family history or the defect can be attributed to disease *in utero* (e.g. maternal rubella). Sometimes there are co-existing congenital abnormalities, as in the Treacher–Collins syndrome (Figs. 9.1 and 9.2). Some patients

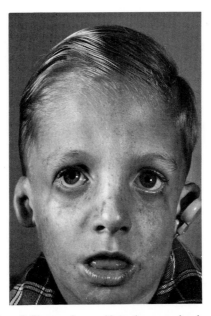

Fig. 9.1   Treacher–Collins syndrome. Note the poor development of the cheek bones, producing an oblique orbit and drooping of the lower lid. There may be atresia of the external canal or microtia. Malformations of the middle ear and ossicles are common. (Reproduced by kind permission of The Royal National Throat, Nose and Ear Hospital, Gray's Inn Rd, London WC1X.)

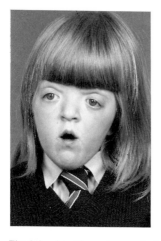 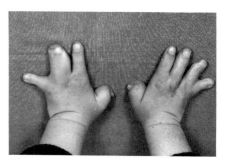

Fig. 9.2 Apert's syndrome. As in Treacher–Collins there is underdevelopment of the cheek bone: there are also defects of the hands and feet.

Abnormalities of bone or connective tissue can cause a conductive loss or SNHL by distorting the normal anatomy of the external, middle or internal ear or of the internal auditory meatus.

present with sensorineural hearing loss arising in adult life, in whom no cause for the deafness can be found. Such cases have been labelled as 'congenital deafness of late onset' (an abuse of the word congenital).

It is beyond the scope of this book to describe all these congenital abnormalities and the interested reader is advised to consult the bibliography.

TRAUMA

In addition to the types of fractures referred to in the previous chapter, less commonly, fractures of the temporal bone as a result of head injury may damage the labyrinth and its nervous connections. This produces immediate, permanent, total loss of hearing and labyrinthine failure. The accompanying facial nerve is also damaged (see Chapter 10).

MENIERE'S DISEASE
(IDIOPATHIC ENDOLYMPHATIC HYDROPS)

This condition is characterized by a combination of three features: cochlear deafness, vertigo and tinnitus. Audiograms taken at three-monthly intervals may show that deafness fluctuates markedly (e.g. over 30–40 dB range) particularly in the early stages of the disease. Recruitment and distortion of sound are troublesome features. The vertigo is episodic lasting for several hours, with associated vomiting, and at its worst the patient has to lie down. This is the so-called 'attack of Meniere's'. However, there is generally a warning which the patient recognizes and most patients with Meniere's can safely be allowed to drive a motor vehicle. If a patient falls over because of vertigo, it is not likely to be due to Meniere's disease. The attacks come on at varying and unpredictable intervals. Between attacks, particularly in the later stages, there may be a persistent feeling of unsteadiness and uncertainty of balance. The tinnitus is often low-pitched, it may become louder during the attack and there may be a feeling of fullness in the affected ear. The disease in this defined form is uncommon.

The condition may begin at almost any age with a peak incidence in the 30–50 year old age group. It runs a course over a few decades with gradually increasing deafness. Initially it affects one ear but in 25% of patients the other ear is eventually affected. Histological examination shows that the membranous labyrinth is distended, that is, there is an increase in the endolymph at the expense of the perilymph, and the organ of Corti degenerates.

Medical treatment is aimed at reducing the volume of endolymph (diuretics and low salt diets have been given) and at suppressing the attacks of vertigo with labyrinthine sedatives. Current surgical treatment attempts to drain off the excess endolymph either by decompressing the endolymphatic sac, or by creating a fistula between the endolymph and perilymph. If the severity of the vertiginous symptoms justifies it and the hearing is good, the vestibular nerves may be divided via the middle or posterior cranial fossa—if symptoms persist, or if there is not useful hearing, the labyrinth may be destroyed. In any case, because the course of the disease is so variable, it is possible neither to predict the result of conservative treatment nor to evaluate it—a large majority of patients with Meniere's report improvement on placebo. The nursing care required before and after surgery is described in Chapter 8.

OTHER CONDITIONS

Spread of infection from chronic suppurative otitis media into the labyrinth (e.g. via erosion of the lateral semicircular canal) produces labyrinthitis, with vertigo—further spread of the process through the labyrinth causes labyrinthine failure and total ipsilateral deafness.

Secondary syphilis may produce labyrinthitis with vertigo. Deafness may be a later result of acquired syphilis or may be due to congenital syphilis.

The only neoplastic condition of importance to be considered is the tumour of the VIII nerve. This neuroma usually affects the coverings of the vestibular part of the VIII nerve and as it grows, produces sensorineural deafness. All unexplained cases of unilateral sensorineural hearing loss need careful investigation if this tumour is not to be missed. There are often symptoms of labyrinthine disturbance and the caloric test almost always shows diminished ipsilateral function. In more advanced cases, the facial nerve is affected. Untreated the condition progresses, generally very slowly over years, with eventual involvement of the lower cranial nerves and cerebellar and brainstem compression. X-rays show enlargement of the internal auditory canal in almost all cases; but if these are normal and there is a high degree of suspicion, tomography, CT scanning and contrast studies may be necessary. Treatment is by surgical excision of the tumour and in early cases, the facial nerve may be spared.

A basis for the ENT aspects of nursing care before and after excision is described in Chapter 8, but it is usual for these patients to be nursed in a neurosurgical unit because of the particular nature of the care required.

10 Facial Nerve Paralysis

The facial nerve is of great importance to otologists, anatomically because it runs a complicated course through the temporal bone, and functionally because if it fails to conduct nerve impulses, facial expressions, a most important part of our interpersonal relationships, are distorted.

CAUSES OF FACIAL NERVE PARALYSIS

Trauma

Within the bone the VII nerve is vulnerable to damage from head injury where there is a fracture of the temporal bone. Two types of temporal bone fracture have been described.

1   Longitudinal: in the long axis of the temporal bone, such a fracture often being in continuity with a fissure fracture of the side of the skull.
2   Transverse: at right angles to the above, often part of an injury to the skull base.

The facial nerve is also liable to damage when the surgeon is carrying out a mastoidectomy or removing an acoustic neuroma. Surrounding disease which has to be removed may be immediately adjacent to the nerve and an accurate knowledge of its course is essential to safe surgery; following these operations the facial nerve function should therefore be checked.

Infection

The VII nerve may be involved from the destructive process of cholesteatoma in the absence of gross infection, though this is unusual even with extensive disease; CSOM associated with facial paralysis seriously raises the possibility of carcinoma or tuberculosis involving the middle ear. The facial nerve is particularly liable to be involved in spread of infection from the middle ear in those cases where it is not completely covered by bone. (The commonest site for this bony dehiscence is just above the oval window.)

Tumours

Beyond the temporal bone, the facial nerve may be involved in a carcinoma of the parotid gland. Tumours of the VII nerve producing paralysis are rare, but the nerve may be involved by an adjacent tumour of the VIII nerve as they pass together in the internal auditory meatus. A gradually progressive paralysis must be regarded as being caused by a neoplasm until proven otherwise.

Idiopathic

In the majority of cases of facial palsy, no definite cause can be found. These are generally labelled Bell's Palsy. This condition presents with an acute onset of paralysis, and except in a few cases where there is some pain in the region of the ear, it is completely painless. Bilateral occurrence is rare. In about 90% of patients there is complete or almost complete recovery, generally within 6–12 weeks. The paralysis may well be due to a viral neuritis. Some authorities believed the resulting oedema of the nerve as it passed through the temporal bone caused it to become devitalized. This led in some places to a vogue for facial nerve decompression (see p. 90).

ASSESSMENT

Careful examination of the patient in a good light is essential, as if even a flicker of movement is detected the nerve must be in continuity, and surgical interference may not be helpful. The patient should be asked to raise the eyebrows, screw up the eyes, puff out the cheeks, open the lips widely and, where it is important to record progress, photographs of the face should be taken in standard positions (Fig. 10.1).

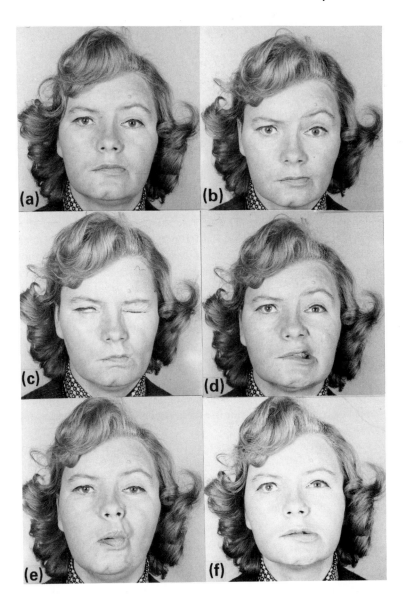

Fig. 10.1 Facial palsy. A record of facial movements is of value in assessing progress. Photographs are taken of the face in a variety of standard expressions. (a) At rest; (b) raising the eyebrows; (c) closing the eyes tightly; (d) showing the teeth; (e) whistling; (f) smiling.

TREATMENT

When the paralysis is due to a progressive infection or destructive disease, surgical treatment to eradicate the disease where possible is the first step.

If it is certain that the continuity of the nerve has been interrupted, continuity should be restored either by mobilization and repair or by nerve grafting; donor nerves commonly include the great auricular nerve, available from the operation field, and a nerve from the lower leg (sural nerve). Alternatively, the hypoglossal nerve (which supplies the ipsilateral half of the muscles of the tongue) can be divided and its proximal end joined to the distal part of the facial nerve. These techniques are only applicable if the facial muscles are capable of functioning; if they have been paralysed too long (about 2 years) they become fibrotic and cannot contract—in this case plastic procedures using muscle grafts or fascial slings can be attempted. None of these operations gives a perfect result but the improvement can be very worthwhile. It will be at least 6 months before improvement in facial muscle movement is evident.

Conversely, if it is certain that the nerve has not been interrupted an expectant policy should probably be adopted. There is no convincing evidence that for Bell's Palsy decompression of the nerve in the mastoid bone has any beneficial effect, and though steroids are often given, their effect on the final recovery is far from clear.

There is an intermediate group of cases due to trauma in which the outcome is initially less certain. Because prolonged paralysis of the muscle leads to irreversible changes, surgery may be advisable if it seems that the prognosis is otherwise poor. Various electrical tests may be helpful in making this decision.

PRE-OPERATIVE CARE

The general physical and psychological care is outlined in Chapter 1. A post aural approach is used so the area behind the pinna needs to be free from hair, as will the leg if a nerve graft is to be taken from this area.

POSTOPERATIVE CARE

On return to the ward the patient is initially nursed on the unaffected side for the reasons given in Chapter 8. When able to move around he should be helped into the most comfortable position. Observations of vital signs, the wound and care of the pressure bandage are described in Chapter 8.

Fluid balance records are maintained until any intravenous infusion is removed and the intake by mouth is adequate. Nausea is often a problem for 24 hours following surgery; anti-emetics will be required, and analgesia for the relief of pain.

Postoperative Care in Nerve Graft Patients

When a nerve graft has been taken from a leg, this leg should not bear weight for 48 hours. During this time the leg is supported on a stool when the patient is sitting out of bed. If a bathroom is nearby, the patient can usually hop to the toilet if supported by two nurses, otherwise he can be taken by wheelchair or a commode can be used. A firm dressing and bandage is applied to the leg in the operating theatre; these are removed and a light dressing applied approximately 24 hours later.

GENERAL NURSING CARE FOR FACIAL NERVE PARALYSIS

Some patients suffering from facial nerve paralysis are not admitted into hospital. The care of a person suffering from Bell's Palsy may be shared by the GP, ENT specialist, community nurse and possibly a physiotherapist.

Facial nerve paralysis may be rapid or gradual in onset depending on the cause. A person first finding his face paralysed when seeing it in a mirror in the morning may be fearful he has suffered a stroke or has a brain tumour. It can take a considerable amount of careful explanation before these fears are allayed. Facial nerve paralysis is disfiguring; it cannot be hidden and it can cause a great deal of mental anguish. The patient will need much psychological care and support especially if the prognosis for recovery is poor. The age of the patient is irrelevant; the elderly do not find facial disfigurement any easier to accept than the young.

As a temporary measure, facial appearance can be improved by attaching a hook to the upper teeth or dentures which will lift up the corner of the mouth. A plumper to fill out the cheek may be held in place by the same method.

Loss of Tears and Taste

There may be unilateral loss of lacrimation and/or taste depending upon the site of the lesion. The eye cannot close when there is a complete palsy; this combined with lack of tears leaves the cornea unprotected. Artificial tear drops can be used several times daily. Dryness and irritation are more marked when central heating is in use. Attempts to humidify a room with bowls of water near the heaters can sometimes be helpful. When going outdoors into a strong wind the eye should be protected by taping it closed. For long term protection spectacles fitted with side shields are useful. If recovery is doubtful or delayed a temporary or permanent tarsorrhaphy can be performed. The eye may need to be irrigated with sterile normal saline at body temperature to remove any dust or debris.

In the absence of blinking, tears are no longer moved across the eye to the lacrimal sac and spill onto the face (epiphora). The tendency to keep wiping tears away with a handkerchief may be irresistible and unfortunately can cause corneal injury and conjunctivitis. Drainage of tears will improve as nerve function and muscle movement return.

The sense of taste is often affected owing to involvement of the chorda tympani nerve (see Chapter 7). There is little that can be done about this except to give an explanation to the patient and ensure an adequate supply of condiments and sauces is available to add to the taste of his food.

Loss of Muscle Tone

Food collects between the paralysed buccinator (cheek) muscle and gums on the affected side, and so eating becomes a problem. Drinking can be embarrassing as fluid and saliva tend to trickle out of the corner of the mouth on the paralysed side. It is necessary to rinse out the mouth after meals to remove any particles of food trapped between cheek, gum and teeth.

If the physiotherapist is involved the patient may be asked to exercise the facial muscles once or twice each day. This mainly involves producing vowel sounds. A mirror and privacy should be provided so that the patient can see his face whilst doing the exercises. Initially the patient will benefit from the presence of a nurse to give support and encouragement. There is no therapeutic value in gently massaging the sagging muscles in an upwards direction from chin to forehead, but it can be of psychological value in some patients. These exercises and chewing on the affected side can help maintain muscle tone until regeneration of the nerve occurs and voluntary movements return; they will not prevent atrophy if regeneration does not occur.

The nasal muscles are affected in facial palsy and the effectiveness of sniffing can be reduced; mucous secretions can thus trickle from the nasal cavity on to the upper lip. Wiping away these secretions can make the surrounding skin quite inflamed and it will require protection with a barrier cream or a preparation such as yellow soft paraffin.

Ramsey Hunt's Syndrome

In Ramsey Hunt's syndrome (Herpes zoster oticus) facial palsy is accompanied by severe pain which will require analgesia. Vertigo, tinnitus and a sensorineural hearing loss may also be present. The patient feels quite debilitated at first and will require complete bed rest for several days. A soothing lotion such as calamine may be applied to the herpetic vesicles which erupt around the pinna, external auditory canal and tympanic membrane.

Recovery

If there is poor recovery the patient may be left with embarrassing problems such as 'crocodile tears' and/or associated movements. Both are due to the misdirection of recovering nerve fibres. When associated movements are present eyelid movements produce an involuntary movement of the mouth, and vice versa. Crocodile tears when the patient eats are due to the re-routed nerve fibres stimulating the lacrimal gland. Surgical section of the nerve supplying the gland will stop the flow of tears.

Even when the prognosis is good, recovery can take many months. During this time the patient has to live with the various problems described which can cause a great deal of unhappiness.

The hospital stay may be short, but nurses working in the community, general practice and OPD will come into contact with these patients and they should have a sympathetic understanding of the difficulties that facial nerve paralysis can cause.

11 Vertigo and Tinnitus

VERTIGO

Although the word vertigo is from the Latin *vertere*, to turn, it is now less strictly used and refers to any hallucination of movement. The sensation of movement and balance in health depends on agreement of the sensory input from various sensory organs (see Chapter 3); vertigo occurs if there is 'disagreement'. Vertigo which is due to a vestibular (labyrinthine*) disorder usually has a rotatory quality, but general vague feelings of unsteadiness or imbalance and staggering also occur. The symptom is often alarming with a strong emotional component and the patient may find it difficult to describe the symptoms. The majority of patients attending an ENT outpatient clinic with vertigo do not have a demonstrable labyrinthine disorder. Fortunately, the patterns of disease caused by such a disorder are on the whole characteristic and distinct. A vestibular disorder may be due to a lesion in the vestibular labyrinth, vestibular nerve or vestibular nuclei. Where a diagnosis can be made, the commonest is Meniere's disease (see Chapter 8).

Causes Due to Disease within the Bony Labyrinth

Benign Positional Vertigo

This is characterized by transitory attacks of vertigo brought on by changes in head position, for example lying down, turning over in bed or looking upwards. The episodes last several seconds, but are very dramatic. The condition is generally self-limiting, but

---

*Although it is correct to talk of the bony labyrinth as defined in Chapter 2, otologists commonly use the term 'labyrinthine' when referring to the aspects of inner ear function relating to balance and movement.

some patients have troublesome symptoms for years. The mechanism and aetiology are not fully understood, but some patients have had a mastoidectomy years previously, and others have had a recent head injury with loss of consciousness. A patient may have been admitted to hospital because of the injury and the vertigo may first occur while convalescing at home. The patient fears to put his head in the positions which provoke the attacks and learns in time to avoid them. Generally this condition is easily diagnosed from the history and from eliciting benign positional nystagmus (see Chapter 5). Perhaps the best treatment for this condition is Cooksey–Cawthorne head and neck exercises.

Epidemic Labyrinthitis

Epidemic labyrinthitis is a poor name for another dramatic disease, as there is little evidence that the adjective 'epidemic' is relevant. The history and progress are again characteristic. The patient, generally a young adult, wakes up in the morning feeling acutely giddy, as though he is being tipped out of bed. There is acute nausea and vomiting, but the patient is too dizzy to walk to the toilet and may scramble about on hands and knees. The condition improves over several hours and vertigo is then only induced by movement. Within a few days he feels quite well again. The disease is thought to be due to a viral infection involving the vestibular nucleus, and it may follow a recent cold.

Other texts mention 'vestibular neuronitis' but there is not general agreement as to what this is; some cases appear to be what is labelled here as epidemic labyrinthitis.

Infective Labyrinthitis

Infective labyrinthitis is suspected clinically in a patient with CSOM who develops vertigo as a new symptom (see p. 67), and this is an indication for early operative treatment.

Causes Due to Disease beyond the Bony Labyrinth

Non-labyrinthine causes of vertigo include diseases of the cerebellum and brain stem, anaemia, raised intracranial tension, postural hypotension and cardiac dysrhythmias, but many cases have no demonstrable cause and are presumably due to transient ischaemia.

Cerebro-vascular Accidents

Cerebro-vascular accidents, in particular thrombosis of the posterior inferior cerebellar artery, produce vertigo but other nerve centres are also involved, usually with impairment of pharyngeal movement, causing dysphagia.

Episodic Ischaemia

Episodic ischaemia of the brain stem and vestibular nuclei may precipitate attacks of acute vertigo which also may be related to posture or movement of the neck.

Vestibular Failure

In acute vestibular failure there is profound vertigo, with the patient unable to stand unaided, and marked spontaneous nystagmus. This may take several weeks to moderate. It may follow head injury but in most cases is presumably due to a vascular accident involving the vestibular nerve and its connections.

Other Causes of Vertigo

Vestibular function can also be affected by therapeutic drugs (particularly streptomycin and dihydrostreptomycin); by secondary syphilis; by tumour of the VIII nerve, and by a viral infection of the geniculate ganglion. Viral infections can probably produce a spectrum of disorders involving the ear, including bullous myringitis (in which there are clear or blood filled vesicles on the tympanic membrane); facial nerve palsy; sensorineural hearing loss; the Ramsey Hunt syndrome (see Chapter 9), and even encephalitis. Transient vertigo in the young adult may be an early manifestation of multiple sclerosis.

Care of a person suffering from vertigo is described in Chapter 8.

TINNITUS

Tinnitus is the sensation of sound arising in the head. It varies in different patients from the trivial to a symptom which dominates the waking life, becoming unbearable, and persons so afflicted may complain they cannot live with it and contemplate or commit suicide. The true incidence is not known, but in approximately 1 million of the British population it is sufficiently bad to significantly affect the enjoyment of life.

In a small proportion, the noise can be heard by another observer (though amplification may be necessary). This type is called *objective tinnitus*. Such noise is often in time with the heart beat, in which case it is probably due to turbulent blood flow. Stereo phonocraniography and X-rays may help to localize the lesion, but it must be remembered that angiography is not without risk. Another cause is intermittent contraction of palatal or middle ear muscles, which produces an irregular clicking.

In the vast majority no noise can be heard objectively—it is a disorder of auditory function and most of these patients have some deafness. The saddest cases are those with tinnitus together with profound or total deafness. Approximately 30% of patients have normal hearing as determined by pure tone audiometry. Many drugs have been reported as causing tinnitus. Important ones include quinine, streptomycin, salicylates and aminoglycoside antibiotics. In the examination of the patient the cause of any associated deafness is sought. Speech audiometry and X-rays of the internal auditory meatus may be requested where there is clinical suspicion of an acoustic neuroma.

Generally, no treatable cause is found. Even where there is associated conductive hearing loss, middle ear surgery, while it may improve the hearing, often does not improve the tinnitus and may make it worse.

Where applicable, a hearing aid often gives relief from tinnitus. In the last few years tinnitus maskers (similar in appearance to a behind the ear hearing aid) have become available and are undergoing careful evaluation in Britain at present. These appear to help a significant proportion of patients who are not too deaf. For those with depression, psychotherapy and antidepressants are useful. Drugs which in some cases take away the tinnitus are also being studied but those available are, as yet, not without side-effects. Most patients referred are able to accept the symptom once they have been reassured that there is no sinister cause.

USEFUL ADDRESSES FOR SELF HELP
GROUPS AND INFORMATION

British Tinnitus Association,
Royal National Institute for the Deaf,
105 Gower Street,
London WC1E 6AH; *or*
9a Clairmont Gardens,
Glasgow G3 47W.

12 Deafness

Although deafness used to be considered a lesser disability than blindness, its seriousness and its effect on life are still not sufficiently realized by the public at large. Deaf people may be thought foolish, and being unable to join in the fun of friendly conversation, they may become suspicious and hostile, and feel they are being ridiculed. For the child, deafness is even more serious as language development depends on the ability to hear. With minor degrees of deafness the child misses some of the auditory input and the intense learning phase of early life is less effective.

Conductive deafness is due to attenuation of sound vibrations reaching the inner ear fluid. Causes include:
1 Meatal atresia.
2 Wax filling the external canal.
3 Occlusion of the meatus from oedema (e.g. by otitis externa).
4 Perforation or scarring of the tympanic membrane.
5 A rigid tympanic membrane owing to infiltration by tympano-sclerosis (chalk).
6 Middle ear effusion (particularly 'glue').
7 Discontinuity of the ossicular chain from trauma, congenital malformation or from bony necrosis.
8 Fixation of the ossicles, for example of the incus and malleus by tympanosclerosis, or of the stapes by otosclerosis.

Perceptive or sensorineural deafness is due to a defect of the cochlea (cochlear deafness) or its nervous connections (retro-cochlear deafness). Defects of the cochlea include:
1 Damage from direct trauma (head injury).
2 Loss of hair cells from acoustic trauma, noise induced hearing loss, or ototoxic drugs.
3 Meniere's disease (endolymphatic hydrops). See Chapter 9.

4 Congenital malformation of the cochlea and organ of Corti.
5 Ischaemic damage from poor blood supply.

Retrocochlear deafness results from impairment of the conduction from the cochlea along the VIII nerve. The most important cause is VIII nerve tumour, but impairment of nerve conduction may be a feature of presbyacusis. In these conditions there is greater loss of speech discrimination than would be expected from the pure tone audiogram.

PRESBYACUSIS

There is increasing deafness with advancing years, at least in the Western civilization. Audiometrically this may initially appear as a bilateral symptomless high tone sensorineural hearing loss, the lower tones becoming gradually involved but degeneration of neural tissue may produce loss of intelligibility and understanding.

NOISE INDUCED HEARING LOSS (NIHL)
(Table 12.1)

A single exposure to a sufficiently loud sound (e.g. an explosion) may cause permanent profound deafness. More commonly this type of injury causes temporary deafness, together with tinnitus which tends to last longer than the deafness. Repeated noise, for example from weapon firing or prolonged noise from machinery, has a cumulative effect producing progressive deafness over the years. NIHL has now become recognized as an industrial disease in certain occupations and may attract compensation.

On the other hand employers are under a legal obligation to care properly for their workforce and if strict standards of noise exposure, in terms of loudness and duration (currently 90 dB(A) for an 8 hour working day) are exceeded then they are liable to prosecution unless they provide adequate protection (e.g. ear plugs or muffs) and instruct workers in its use. Several large firms now carry out monitoring audiometry (see Chapter 5) so that if damage occurs it can be detected early, even before the worker is aware of any hearing loss. The earliest change is seen on the pure tone audiogram as a dip at 4 kHz. With further exposure this deepens and adjacent frequencies are progressively involved.

Table 12.1.   Decibels produced by common sound sources.

Decibel	Sound situation or source
0	Silence; threshold of hearing
10	Rustling paper
20	Whispering
30	Ticking watch positioned 1 m from the ear
40	Quiet room
50	Quiet conversation
60	Normal conversation
70	Loud conversation
80	Heavy traffic
90	Engineering workshop
100	Boilermakers shop
110	Road drill
120	Jet engine
130	Threshold of pain/discomfort
140	Shotgun blast (causing pain and perforation of the tympanic membrane)

Microscopically, degeneration of the outer hair cells of the cochlea is seen, occurring maximally in the basal turn. Similar microscopic cochlear damage is produced by ototoxic drugs and in conditions where the blood supply is thought to be inadequate (presbyacusis, diabetes or hyperlipoproteinaemia). Clinically, patients find difficulty in understanding speech (because the consonants are complex high frequency sounds) though they can hear music. There is also a stage where, because of the outer hair cell loss, quiet sounds are not heard while with the preservation of the inner hair cells the appreciation of loud sounds as being loud is retained. This leads to an apparent paradox with the patient not hearing quiet sounds and then with increasing loudness of the sound the patient suddenly hears it very loudly. This phenomenon is *recruitment* (see Chapter 5) and is seen in the deaf person who exclaims 'don't shout, I'm not deaf' or who shudders when a door bangs. This is an oversimplification of recruitment; the interested reader is referred to the bibliography.

CONGENITAL DEAFNESS

Congenital deafness may be due to genetic causes (i.e. a defect of the embryo) or to foetal damage during pregnancy. Various types of embryonic defects of the cochlea are described and given eponyms; some are associated with other congenital defects, particularly of the external ear. An important cause of foetal damage producing deafness is maternal rubella. Foetal hypoxia during parturition or kernicterus in the early postnatal period may damage the cochlear nuclei in the brain stem producing deafness.

Treatment of Congenital Deafness

It is important to recognize the profoundly deaf baby as soon as possible and babies known to be 'at risk' (for example from a family history of hereditary deafness, from complications at parturition or from maternal rubella), should be given particular attention. The normal neonate executes a 'startle reflex' in response to a loud sound (e.g. a hand clap). Various screening tests are described for the older baby and the reader is referred to the bibliography. Commonly, even in the profoundly deaf child there are some sounds which the child can hear provided amplification is sufficient, and these can be utilized in the education of the child. Thorough testing needs the facilities of a child assessment centre, and in considering the child with other handicaps (e.g. mental or neurological) the use of evoked response audiometry with the child anaesthetized can be invaluable. The imperative need is for the child to learn to communicate and for the profoundly deaf there is controversy as to whether it is better for the child to learn to speak or to learn a sign language which may be quicker and easier for him. Special facilities exist in schools for the deaf.

Hearing impairment acquired after speech has developed, termed *post-lingual deafness*, may still be serious but is less so as the individual has already learned to communicate.

COMMUNICATING WITH THE HEARING IMPAIRED PERSON

The nurse should first enquire, and record, whether the hearing impaired person uses lip-reading, finger spelling or sign language.

Unilateral Deafness

Where there is a useful amount of hearing in one ear good communication can be maintained by the person turning his head slightly so that the better ear is towards the person who is talking. This allows maximum use of the hearing ear without losing sight of the other person's face.

Lip-reading

The following points should be observed:
1   Only talk to the patient when you are facing him and he can see your face in a good light.
2   Do not cover or touch your lips when talking to the patient.
3   Do not shout. Shouting distorts the face making lip-reading more difficult, and can cause discomfort to the patient who has recruitment.
4   Talk at a slightly slower rate than normal with the voice slightly raised.
5   Lip movements should be well formed, but not exaggerated as this also causes distortion of the face.
6   Remember that the hearing impaired person supplements what is heard, and gained from lip-reading, with other forms of non-verbal communication such as eye contact, hand movements, and facial expressions.

Finger Spelling and Sign Language

In finger spelling each letter of the alphabet is represented by a particular position of the fingers and words are built up letter by letter. It is quite easy to learn and like most manual skills, practice makes perfect.

Sign language is the use of certain signs for words and phrases. It is quicker than using finger spelling, but as it is more complicated it will take longer to learn. As each country has some of its own signs it is of limited help in communicating with deaf people from other countries.

Handwriting

Handwriting is normally used only as a last resort. Obviously its use is not possible if the patient is illiterate or has very poor vision.

Hearing Aids

All electrical hearing aids have three major parts: a microphone which picks up the sound, an amplifier which makes the sound

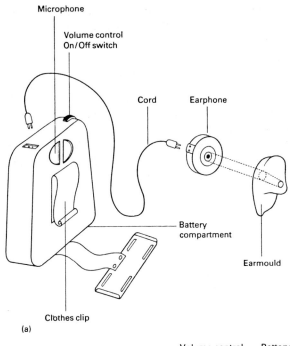

Microphone

Volume control
On/Off switch

Cord

Earphone

Battery
compartment

Earmould

Clothes clip

(a)

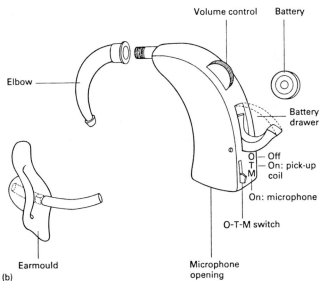

Volume control

Battery

Elbow

Battery
drawer

O — Off
T — On: pick-up
M   coil

On: microphone

O-T-M switch

Earmould

Microphone
opening

(b)

Fig. 12.1 (a) Body worn hearing aid, type OL56; (b) behind the ear hearing aid, type BE11.

louder and is powered by batteries, and an earpiece or receiver which delivers the sound to the ear via an earmould.

There are two types of electrical hearing aid (Fig. 12.1) available on the NHS: body worn aids (BW series) and behind the ear aids (BE series).

Body worn aids have the microphone, amplifier and battery in a case which is worn on the body. A cord runs from this case connecting it to the receiver and earmould in the ear. The best position for the aid is near the centre of the chest. It can be clipped onto clothing, contained within a purse-like bag or suspended from a cord around the neck. Young active children need something stronger and more stable than a small bag, and special harnesses which can be used for one or two body worn aids are available for their use. The microphone must always be uncovered and face outwards.

Behind the ear aids have all the parts in a small case that fits snugly behind the ear. Sound is carried into the earmould by a small piece of plastic tubing. The small size of these aids, their hidden position and lack of a trailing wire makes them popular.

In addition, in-the-ear aids and spectacle aids (with the components built into a spectacle arm) may be purchased from a private hearing aid dispenser, and although costly, they can appear very attractive for aesthetic reasons.

Hearing aids are worthwhile for the child with recurrent glue ear or when such a child is under the care of a doctor who prefers conservative management of these children. They are particularly helpful for patients with a conductive hearing loss. They are also helpful in patients with a sensorineural hearing loss, although recruitment or predominantly high tone loss present special problems. Aids are probably not worthwhile where speech discrimination is poor.

Testing Aids

There are several reasons why a hearing aid may not work and ENT wards and departments should have available a selection of cords, batteries and pieces of plastic tubing which can be used to replace worn parts when there is no Hearing Aid Centre open nearby.

To test if a BW aid is working, take the earmould off the receiver, turn the volume control to maximum and place the receiver about a foot from the front of a microphone. If the aid is working there should be a high pitched whistling sound (feedback). To test if a BE aid is working, switch the aid on (M for microphone position) turn the volume control to maximum and cup the aid in the palm of the hand. Again, 'feedback' should be heard.

Functional Problems

Hearing aids are steadily improving, and will continue to do so. However, they are not without problems, particularly if the ear discharges from time to time, or is prone to otitis externa—in these circumstances it may be helpful to use a bone conducting aid in which the earphone, resting behind the ear, transmits sound via the mastoid bone. In addition, the tiny controls may be difficult for an arthritic hand to adjust. The following are fairly common hearing aid problems:

1 The battery may be exhausted, and a new battery should be tried before taking any other steps. NHS aids and batteries are marked to assist in correct placement of batteries, but all NHS aids can be fitted with ordinary commercial batteries of the correct size and power.

2 The earmould must be very comfortable and a snug fit. It should not be too loose or too tight or it will rub against the skin, causing discomfort, itching and irritation. It can get blocked with wax and debris and should be detached from the aid and washed in warm soapy water. It must be absolutely dry before being replaced on the aid.

3 The cord on a BW aid can crack. If this has happened it will need to be replaced.

4 The flexible plastic tube which connects the earmould to the rigid plastic tube on BE models may kink and block the passage of sound or it may crack and allow sound to escape. It can quite easily be removed and replaced.

5 If the hearing aid whistles when it is in the patient's ear the noise is due to sound escaping from the ear and producing feedback. This happens when the earmould is too loose and not fitting properly. Before arranging for the suply of a new one, check that the existing mould is being fitted into the ear correctly, and that there is not an accumulation of wax preventing this.

A hearing aid is not a cure for deafness. It will only amplify the sound that reaches it and it is important to remember that most users supplement what is being heard by lip-reading.

Other Types of Aid

Ear trumpets, 'banjos', auricles and speaking tubes are still available on the NHS. As they have no finger controls or batteries that need changing they still have a place, usually for the elderly.

A communicator (Fig. 12.2) is a very useful piece of equipment for most areas and situations both in and out of hospital. It is battery operated, simple to use and quite cheap.

Radio and Television Aids

Those with a hearing loss may find it impossible to hear a television or radio adequately whilst they are in hospital unless special provisions are made. These patients may have been accustomed to turning the volume up to a level that was acceptable in their own home with family and friends, but which is unacceptable in a hospital!

Adaptors are available which make it unnecessary for the volume to be turned up so high that it disturbs others and is

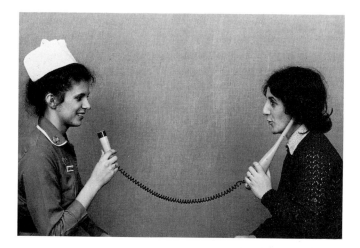

Fig. 12.2 The battery operated communicator in use. The nurse speaks into the microphone end; the other end has a handle which is long enough for the patient to hold comfortably whilst keeping the sound source against her ear.

embarrassing. These adaptors can also make it possible for a better quality of sound to be obtained. One such adaptor consists of a separate earphone which is connected to the set and used instead of a hearing aid. The other adaptor available makes use of what is known as the Loop system. In this system a loop of wire is placed round a room and connected to the loudspeaker terminals inside a television or radio set. Some BE aids have a pick up coil inside the aid through which the programme can then be heard. The pick up position on the switch is usually marked with a T (Fig. 12.1).

Neither of these adaptors is expensive, indeed many people use them in their own home and it is recommended that they are available in any hospital area where there is likely to be a need for them.

INFORMATION SOURCES

Royal National Institute for the Deaf,
105 Gower Street, London WC1E 6AH; *or*
9a Clairmont Gardens, Glasgow G3 7LW.

National Deaf Children's Society,
45 Hereford Road, London W2 3DA.

British Association of Hard of Hearing,
6 Great James Street, London WC1 3DA.

British Deaf Association,
38 Victoria Place, Carlisle CA1 1HU.

Breakthrough Trust,
The Link Room,
Charles W. Gillett Centre,
Selly Oak Colleges,
Birmingham B29 6LE.

The Post Office
'Help for the Handicapped' (leaflet)

DHSS
'General Guidance for Hearing Aid Users' (booklet)

Local Education Authorities
Many authorities make provision for lip-reading, finger spelling and sign language instruction.

PART II · THE NOSE

13 Applied Anatomy and Physiology of the Nose and Sinuses

EXTERNAL NOSE

The external nose is pyramidal in shape, and has a bony and cartilaginous framework covered with skin (Fig. 13.1).

The upper part of the framework is formed mainly by the nasal bones. The lower part of the framework consists of the upper lateral cartilages, and the lower lateral (alar) cartilages, each having a medial and lateral crus. The septal cartilage adds support in the midline, its dorsal edge meeting the medial borders of the upper lateral cartilages.

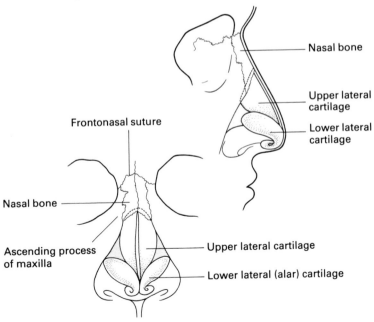

Fig. 13.1   The structure of the nasal pyramid.

NASAL CAVITIES

The nasal septum divides the interior of the nose into two cavities; these open anteriorly via the nares, where they are separated by the columella which is joined to the anterior end of the septum. Posteriorly the nasal cavities communicate with the nasopharynx via the choanae (Fig. 13.2).

The anterior part of each nasal cavity, just within the nares, is termed the nasal vestibule, it is lined with skin and contains hairs (vibrissae). It is bounded posteriorly by the limen nasi, a curved ridge which represents the lower margin of the upper lateral cartilage. The region of the limen is the narrowest part of the nasal air passage, and is sometimes referred to as the nasal valve.

Posterior to the limen, each nasal cavity is lined with mucous membrane. The boundaries of each nasal cavity are outlined below.

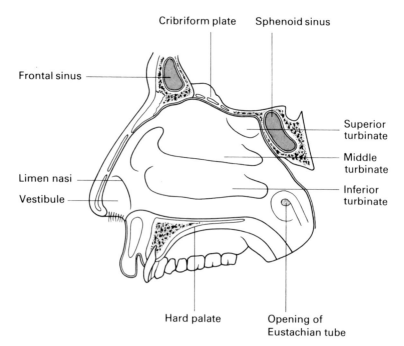

Fig. 13.2   Sagittal section through the right nasal cavity to show its lateral wall.

Boundaries

Floor

The bone of the hard palate, separating the nose from the mouth.

Roof

The cribriform plate of bone, separating the nose from the anterior cranial fossa, through which fibres of the olfactory nerve pass.

Medial Wall

The nasal septum—cartilaginous anteriorly, bony posteriorly.

Lateral Wall

The bony lateral wall separates the nose inferiorly from the maxillary sinus, and superiorly from the cells of the ethmoidal sinus. Attached to the lateral wall are three turbinates (superior, middle and inferior), and under each turbinate is the corresponding meatus. The paranasal sinuses open through ostia into the lateral wall of the nose, and most drain into the middle meatus. The nasolacrimal duct (tear duct) opens into the inferior meatus just beneath the anterior end of the inferior turbinate.

PARANASAL SINUSES

The paranasal sinuses (Fig. 13.3) are air-filled cavities lined with ciliated mucous membrane, lying within the bones of the skull adjacent to the nose. There are four on each side, communicating with the nasal cavities via narrow openings (ostia).

Maxillary Sinus/Antrum

The maxillary sinus or antrum is shaped like a pyramid lying on its side, its base forming the lower part of the lateral wall of the nose, and its apex extending laterally towards the zygoma. Its boundaries are outlined below.

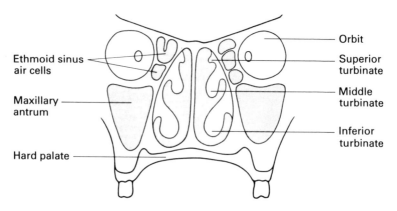

Fig. 13.3   Coronal section through the nose and paranasal sinuses.

Medial

The bony wall separating the sinus from the nasal cavity. Below the inferior turbinate the bone is thin or dehiscent, and this is the site punctured when performing an antral wash-out.

Lateral

The apex extends to the zygomatic process of the maxilla.

Superior

The thin bony roof of the sinus is also the floor of the orbit.

Inferior

The hard palate, and alveolar bone carrying some of the upper teeth.

Anterior

The anterior bony wall separates the sinus from the soft tissues of the cheek.

Posterior

The posterior bony wall intervenes between the sinus and the pterygo-palatine fossa.

The ostium of the maxillary sinus opens into the middle meatus, and is thus situated high up on the medial wall of the antrum, where it is inefficiently placed as a drainage point.

Ethmoid Sinuses/Labyrinth

These consist of a gallery of about ten intercommunicating air cells, sandwiched between the orbit and the nasal cavity, with the anterior cranial fossa above and the maxillary antrum below. The ethmoid cells drain into the middle and superior meatuses.

Frontal Sinus

The frontal sinus lies within the frontal bone, separated from its fellow of the opposite side by a thin bony septum; the soft tissues of the forehead lie anteriorly, the anterior cranial fossa lies posteriorly, and below its floor lie the orbit and ethmoid cells. It drains via the frontonasal duct downwards into the middle meatus.

Sphenoid Sinus

The sphenoid sinus lies within the sphenoid bone, separated from the sinus of the other side by a bony septum; it is situated high up posteriorly in the roof of the nasal cavity, above the choana. The ostium opens above the superior turbinate into the spheno-ethmoidal recess. The sphenoid sinuses, like the frontals, are usually asymmetrical.

ARTERIAL SUPPLY OF THE NOSE AND PARANASAL SINUSES

The arterial supply is derived from branches of both the external and internal carotid arteries. The most important branch of the external carotid artery supplying the nose is the internal maxillary artery, which pursues a serpentine course from lateral to medial

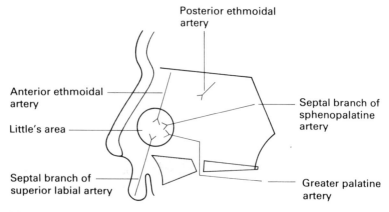

Fig. 13.4 Little's Area and the blood supply of the nasal septum. (Adapted by kind permission from Foxen E. H. M. (1980) *Lecture Notes on Diseases of the Ear, Nose and Throat*, 5th edn., p. 94. Blackwell Scientific Publications, Oxford.)

through the pterygo-palatine fossa, behind the posterior wall of the maxillary antrum where it divides into a number of branches which pass into the nasal cavity. It may be ligated in severe cases of epistaxis, by means of a Caldwell–Luc approach through the maxillary antrum.

The supply from the internal carotid artery is via the anterior and posterior ethmoidal arteries, which arise from the ophthalmic artery and pass through the medial wall of the orbit to reach the nasal cavity. The ethmoidal arteries may be ligated within the orbit to control severe epistaxis, and are approached via a small incision close to the medial canthus of the eye.

A rich anastomosis of vessels termed Kiesselbach's Plexus is situated in Little's Area on the antero-inferior part of the nasal septum (Fig. 13.4). This is said to be the usual site for epistaxis, however the bleeding is often seen to arise from a small vein placed more anteriorly, near the floor of the nose.

NERVE SUPPLY OF THE NOSE

Ordinary sensation is subserved by branches of the fifth cranial nerve; the special sense of smell is derived from branches of the first cranial nerve, which pass from the area of olfactory mucosa in the upper part of the nasal cavity upwards through the cribriform plate to the brain.

MUCOUS MEMBRANE OF THE NOSE AND PARANASAL SINUSES

From the superior turbinate upwards, each nasal cavity is lined with a specialized olfactory mucous membrane which carries nerve endings subserving the sense of smell.

The remainder of each nasal cavity, together with all the paranasal sinuses, is lined with ciliated, columnar, 'respiratory type' epithelium. Goblet cells within this epithelium produce mucus which is continually wafted by the cilia towards the nasopharynx, whence it is swallowed. This ciliary activity is impaired in smokers.

PHYSIOLOGY OF THE NOSE AND PARANASAL SINUSES

The functions of the nose and sinuses are summarized below:
1 'Air conditioning' of inspired air, to protect the lungs.
(a) *Purification* The vibrissae filter out large particles, and smaller particles are trapped in the mucus blanket, swept with it into the nasopharynx and swallowed. Enzymes present in the mucus destroy some bacteria. Large foreign particles are expelled by sneezing.
(b) *Warming* The rich blood supply of the nasal mucosa, and the large surface area afforded by the turbinates, enable inspired air to be efficiently warmed to body temperature by the time it reaches the larynx, even on a cold day.
(c) *Humidification* The nasal secretions almost completely saturate the inspired air with moisture. About 1 litre of fluid is produced by the nose each day, of which approximately 700 ml is used to humidify the inspired air, and the remaining 300 ml is swallowed.
2 Smell.
3 The functions of the sinuses are uncertain. However, various unsubstantiated theories have been proposed, including the following:

(a) a contribution to the air conditioning process,
(b) lightening the skull,
(c) a contribution to vocal resonance,
(d) a contribution to the protection of the brain from facial injury.

14 Clinical Assessment of the Nose

SYMPTOMS

There are several important nasal symptoms, which give useful clues to the diagnosis.

Nasal Obstruction

Nasal obstruction may be constant (and often unilateral) suggesting a mechanical obstruction such as a deviated nasal septum; or it may fluctuate in severity and alternate from side to side, indicating that mucosal swelling is the cause, as in various forms of rhinitis.

Rhinorrhoea

Rhinorrhoea (nasal discharge) may be clear and watery as in allergic rhinitis; or it may be purulent, indicating an infective cause, as in sinusitis. Patients with rhinorrhoea often also complained of mucus trickling from the back of the nose into the throat (post-nasal drip), and they may persistently attempt to clear the mucus from the throat by 'hawking'. A purulent post-nasal drip may give rise to an unpleasant taste.

Sneezing

Sneezing is a well-known symptom of the common cold (a form of infective rhinitis), but bouts of sneezing also occur in other forms of rhinitis, notably the allergic type e.g. hayfever.

Epistaxis

Epistaxis (bleeding from the nose) is dealt with in Chapter 16.

Anosmia

Anosmia or hyposmia (an absent or a reduced sense of smell) accompanies many nasal diseases where air flow to the upper part of the nasal cavities is obstructed.

Headache and Facial Pain

Headache and facial pain may be the result of sinusitis, but there are many other causes which are discussed in Chapter 19.

EXAMINATION

The nose is examined with the aid of a head mirror, which reflects light along the examiner's line of sight, whilst leaving both hands free to manipulate instruments.

Inspection of the Nose

Inspection of the external nose is carried out first, to look for any deformity or skin lesion.

The patency of the nasal airways is next assessed—one nostril is occluded by the examiner's thumb and the patient is asked to sniff in. An alternative technique is to ask the patient to breathe out onto the surface of a Lack's tongue depressor held about 2 cm below the nose, and observe the degree of misting that occurs on the metal surface.

The nasal vestibules are then inspected by turning up the tip of the nose with the examiner's thumb; this technique also provides an adequate view of the lower part of the nasal cavities in children.

Rhinoscopy

Anterior rhinoscopy is carried out using a Thudichum nasal speculum (Fig. 14.1), which normally permits a view of the floor of the nose, the inferior and middle turbinates, and the corresponding part of the septum (Fig. 14.2).

Posterior rhinoscopy is next performed: the tongue is displaced downwards with a Lack's tongue depressor, and a pre-warmed post-nasal mirror is introduced into the oropharynx beyond the

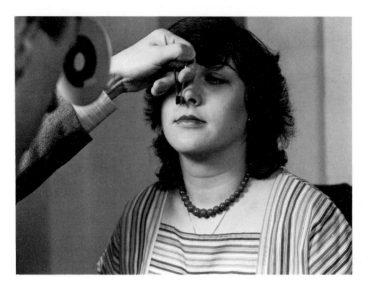

Fig. 14.1 Anterior rhinoscopy.

soft palate. A view is thus obtained of the posterior end of the nasal septum with the choanal openings on each side, through which the posterior ends of the middle and inferior turbinates may be seen. Lateral to the choanal opening on each side lies the orifice of the Eustachian tube, and superiorly the vault of the naso-pharynx comes into view (Fig. 14.3). Examination of the post nasal

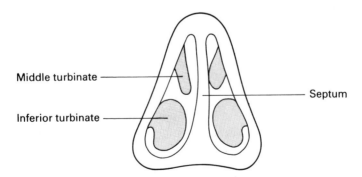

Fig. 14.2 The view obtained by anterior rhinoscopy. (Adapted by kind permission of Foxen E. H. M. (1980) *Lecture Notes on Diseases of the Ear, Nose and Throat*, 5th edn., p. 87. Blackwell Scientific Publications, Oxford.)

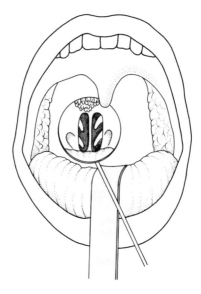

Fig. 14.3   The view obtained by posterior rhinoscopy. (Adapted by kind permission of Foxen E. H. M. (1980) *Lecture Notes on Diseases of the Ear, Nose and Throat*, 5th edn., p. 87. Blackwell Scientific Publications, Oxford.)

space is not easy, and in some individuals it is impossible to obtain an adequate view because of gagging or elevation of the soft palate; in these patients the flexible fibre-optic naso-pharyngo-scope is invaluable (see Chapter 25).

Palpation

The examination of the nose is completed if a nasal neoplasm is suspected, by palpation of the neck for cervical lymph node metastases. It must also be remembered that middle ear disease may be a complication of nasal disorders.

RADIOLOGICAL INVESTIGATIONS

These are of great value in the diagnosis of sinus disease.

Plain Sinus X-rays

Plain sinus X-rays are taken from several different angles, because
no single view will demonstrate all the sinuses adequately. The
following three views are the most commonly employed:

1   Occipitomental (OM) to show the maxillary antra (Fig. 14.4).
2   Occipitofrontal (OF) to show the ethmoid and frontal sinuses.
3   Lateral to show the sphenoid sinus, and the depth of the frontal
sinus.

These plain films can, for example, demonstrate evidence of
infection (mucosal thickening within the sinus, perhaps with a fluid
level), or evidence of a neoplasm with destruction of the sinus
walls, or fractures of the maxilla. Fractures of the nasal bones are
best shown by special supero-inferior (occlusal) and lateral views.

Tomograms

Tomograms may provide additional information, especially in
determining the extent of a neoplasm, and even more detail may
be derived from a computerized tomography scan (CT scan).

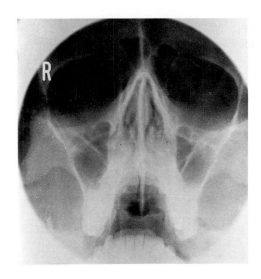

Fig. 14.4   Normal sinus X-ray: occipitomental view.

Antroscopy

When the results of the radiological investigations are equivocal, endoscopic examination of the maxillary sinuses ('antroscopy') may be helpful (see Chapter 25).

15 Nasal Injuries and Deformities

FRACTURE OF THE NASAL BONES

The fracture is generally simple, but may be compound with an overlying laceration in the nasal skin. The nasal bone fragments may be significantly displaced, but often they are not. There may be other associated injuries.

Aetiology

Nasal bone fractures are often the result of an injury sustained in sport, a road traffic accident, or from an assault.

Clinical Features

There is usually epistaxis at the time of injury; there may be a deformity of the nose (flattening or crookedness of the bridge), but this may become obscured by local swelling and bruising. Nasal obstruction may be present due to blood clot, or due to dislocation or haematoma of the septum. Pain is not usually a feature after the initial impact, but the nasal bones are markedly tender, and are sometimes mobile on palpation.

Investigations

X-rays should be taken as they may be important medicolegally, but they seldom influence the course of treatment (Fig. 15.1).

Treatment

An open wound should be cleaned and closed. If there is displacement of the nasal bones, reduction is recommended. Occasionally

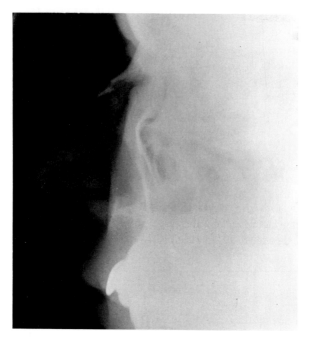

Fig. 15.1 Fractured nasal bones: lateral X-ray.

the patient is seen within 2 hours of injury, and the fracture may be reduced immediately with the aid of some analgesia.

In general, however, the patient is not seen until some hours have elapsed. If by then swelling has obscured the bony landmarks, then the optimum time for manipulation is after the swelling has subsided, but before the bony fragments have become fixed, that is 5–10 days after the injury. Reduction is carried out under general anaesthesia by simple manipulation, or with the aid of a suitable instrument; splintage is often unnecessary, but if the nasal bones are very mobile than a plaster of Paris cast is applied for 7 days. The adhesive tapes holding the plaster in position should not be removed if soiled—clean tapes should be applied over the stained ones. If the cast is dirty it can be whitened with shoe whitener. It is sometimes possible to correct septal fractures and dislocations by manipulation at the same time, but often the result is unsatisfactory and a septoplasty or submucous resection is needed later.

If a patient presents late, months after the injury, union of the bones will have occurred and manipulation will not be successful; a rhinoplasty will be required. Following rhinoplasty there is a variable degree of oedema and bruising around the eyes, which will require gentle bathing. Anterior nasal packs are removed within 24 hours of surgery. The plaster of Paris remains for approximately 7 days before being removed in the OPD. The patient is usually able to go home by the second or third postoperative day. A detailed account of the nursing care is given on p. 134.

FOREIGN BODIES IN THE NOSE

Foreign bodies in the nose are commonly encountered in children; almost any small object may be inserted, but buttons, beads, paper and fragments of foam rubber are amongst the commonest.

Clinical Features

Sometimes the child presents with a clear history of having introduced a foreign body. However, especially in very young children there may be no such history and the complaint is of a unilateral purulent nasal discharge, which is often foul smelling. Examination may reveal the foreign body, but often it is obscured by discharge and mucosal oedema.

Investigations

X-rays are useful in localizing a radio-opaque object such as a ball-bearing.

Treatment

Removal is required. Forceful nose-blowing may expel the object but if this fails it may be possible in a co-operative child to remove an anteriorly placed, clearly visible foreign body using a head mirror, speculum, and forceps or a blunt hook. Extreme care is necessary to prevent posterior displacement, and possible inhalation, of the object. If there is *any* difficulty, or if the child is refractory at the outset, then removal should be performed under general anaesthesia with a pack in the nasopharynx.

Rarely, a foreign body may remain *in situ* unsuspected for years, and gradually acquire a coating of concretions (layers of calcium and magnesium salts) to become a rhinolith. It may then present as a cause of nasal obstruction or discharge in adult life, by which time removal under general anaesthesia may be difficult.

THE DEVIATED NASAL SEPTUM

Few Caucasian adults have a perfectly straight septum; marked deflections, however, may produce symptoms and benefit from correction.

Aetiology

Trauma to the nose is the commonest cause of gross septal deformities. Sometimes, however, buckling of the septum results from an abnormal pattern of growth.

Symptoms

Persistent nasal obstruction predominates. Occasionally an external deformity results, headaches may occur, and recurrent sinus infection may develop due to obstruction of ostial drainage.

Signs

Anterior rhinoscopy readily reveals the septal deformity; this may take the form of a caudal dislocation of the septum at the columella, a deviation of the cartilaginous septum further back, or a bony spur arising far posteriorly. There may be compensatory hypertrophy of a middle or inferior turbinate, filling a concavity left by the distorted septum.

Indications for Surgery

1 Severe obstruction of the nasal airway.
2 Obstruction of sinus drainage resulting in recurrent sinusitis.
3 To obtain access
   (a) to a bleeding point in order to control epistaxis;
   (b) to polyps to permit their adequate removal;
   (c) to the ethmoid and sphenoid sinuses.

Surgical Treatment

If surgery is indicated, then two techniques are available:

1 *Submucous resection* (SMR) is a very satisfactory operation for adults, but should be avoided in children where possible as it may result in depression of the nasal bridge-line (saddle-nose), due to

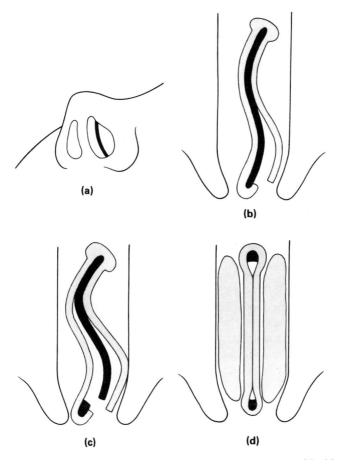

Fig. 15.2 Submucous resection of the septum. (a) The incision; (b), (c), (d) diagrammatic horizontal sections showing the separation of the muco-perichondrium from underlying cartilage and bone (black); in (d), the packs have been inserted. (By kind permission of Foxen E. H. M. (1980) *Lecture Notes on Diseases of the Ear, Nose and Throat*, 5th edn., p. 102. Blackwell Scientific Publications, Oxford.)

interference with the growth of the septum. Under general anaesthesia an incision is made on one side of the septum through the
mucoperichondrium, which is then elevated from the underlying
cartilage (Fig. 15.2). The incision is deepened to divide the
cartilage, and the mucoperichondrial 'flap' is elevated on the other
side as well; deflections and spurs of cartilage and bone can then be
removed from between the two flaps, which are finally allowed to
fall together in the midline. The flaps are supported by nasal packs
which remain *in situ* for 24 hours.
2 *Septoplasty* is a more elaborate technique for straightening the
septum which conserves the cartilage and bone, by re-modelling
and re-positioning it in the midline. It is not suitable for all types of
septal deformity, but can be employed in children, and can be
combined with a rhinoplasty (septorhinoplasty).

Pre-operative Care

There is no specific local preparation unless the surgeon requests
that a vasoconstricting preparation is applied, in the ward area,
before the patient goes to the operating theatre. There are two
methods of applying such a preparation; bilateral nasal packs are
inserted or Moffett's method is used.

A Pre-operative Nasal Pack

The quantity and strength of all drugs used should be prescribed
for each individual. The time for pack insertion is usually 30
minutes before the patient is due to go to theatre. The full
procedure is explained to the patient.

Before premedication is given the nose is sprayed with 4–6 puffs
of the chosen local anaesthetic using a Rogers' spray (Fig. 15.3).
This is necessary to test for unfavourable reaction to the drug and
to anaesthetize the nasal cavity before the pack is inserted. The
pulse is taken before the nose is sprayed and then every 15 minutes
until the patient goes to theatre (see Chapter 28, toxic reaction to
local anaesthetics). The pack is prepared for insertion before the
patient is positioned. As the medication used is not sterile this is
not an aseptic technique but the packing is not handled; sterile
equipment and dressing materials are used, and the hands are
washed. A head mirror and light source should be used during
insertion of the pack. Two lengths of half inch ribbon gauze each

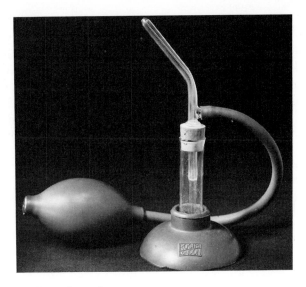

Fig. 15.3 A Rogers' crystal spray.

approximately 1 m long are cut and placed in the vasoconstricting solution. The most commonly used preparation is cocaine 10% (or lignocane 4%) and adrenaline 1:1000 in equal quantities. Using forceps the ribbon gauze is wrung out and laid in folds on a gauze swab in a receiver.

The patient is helped into the tracheostomy position, lying supine with a pillow under the shoulders to extend the neck. If this position is not possible then the patient can sit upright, well supported with pillows. Clothing is protected and a receiver and tissues are at hand. Ask the patient to breathe through his mouth.

The nostril is dilated with a nasal speculum. Using Tilley's forceps the ribbon gauze is introduced into each nasal cavity in folds. Figure 16.1 shows an anterior nasal pack in situ. When both sides are packed the external ends can be tied together, or taped onto the face. Should a reaction to the local anaesthetic occur:
1 Immediately remove the pack.
2 Summon nursing and medical help.
3 Stay with the patient to observe vital signs and airway, and to give reassurance.
4 Reactions are treated symptomatically. Intravenous diazepam may be required.

Moffett's Method

The drugs used and the time for instillation must be prescribed. Instillation is normally requested 30 minutes before the patient is due to go to the operating theatre, or may be performed by the anaesthetist after the patient has been anaesthetized. The same observations for toxic reaction to the drugs used when nasal packing is inserted should be carried out. The generally used quantity of Moffett's method is 5 ml and contains:

2 ml sodium bicarbonate 1%;
2 ml cocaine 8%;
1 ml adrenaline 1:1000.

Lignocaine 4% or cocaine 10% are sometimes used in place of cocaine 8%. The mixture is always prepared immediately prior to installation to prevent deterioration. The procedure is explained to the patient and he is then helped into the supine position with his head hyperextended. The patient is asked to breathe through his mouth throughout the procedure in order to prevent his swallowing or aspirating the solution. Should any solution trickle into the throat he is asked to spit it out, so a receiver and tissues must be at hand.

The solution is drawn into a syringe with an angled blunt needle or a 'kwill' attached. Five drops of the mixture are instilled into each nasal cavity and the head is turned to the left side for 2 minutes, and brought back into the centre. Another 5 drops of the solution are instilled on each side and the head turned to the right; after the third instillation of 5 drops the head is left in the central position. This is continued until there is no solution left.

Five minutes after completion the patient is helped into a more comfortable position.

Post-operative Care

Although a wide variety of materials is used for nasal packing, the presence of a nasal pack will always present some specific nursing problems.

Sitting in a well supported upright position will aid drainage and lessen oedema. Unless there are specific reasons for bed rest, gentle mobilization starts the day after operation.

The patient will have complete nasal obstruction resulting in anosmia and mouth breathing. Regular and thorough oral care is necessary for comfort and oral health. Mouth washes are not an acceptable substitute for brushing the teeth and gums. Anosmia

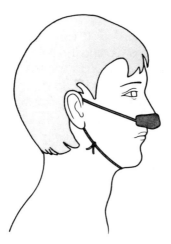

Fig. 15.4 A nasal bolster in position.

will also cause a reduction in taste so the diet must be attractively presented, and preferably of the patient's choice. A wide range of nourishing fluids should be available.

In order to prevent any blood or serous fluid trickling through the packs onto the face a nasal bolster is applied (Fig. 15.4). The tapes are looped over the ears and tied under the chin, not at the back of the head, to prevent undue pressure on the nasal septum. This bolster is changed as it becomes soiled. Whilst in position it can cause problems when drinking from a glass or cup—either it can be removed prior to drinking, or alternatively a straw or spouted feeding cup can be used.

The surgical trauma and presence of the pack will result in the formation of oedema which may cause obstruction of the naso-lacrimal duct and the ostia of the paranasal air sinuses. Epiphora may occur and the overflow of tears is both irritating and uncomfortable, and in these instances the eyes should be bathed regularly. If a secondary sinusitis occurs there may be pyrexia and pain over the affected sinus.

Removal of Anterior Nasal Packs

Anterior nasal packs are removed upon written instructions from the doctor. The removal of small packs is straightforward but, if the packs are large an analgesic or sedative given before their removal may be helpful.

Nasal packs should always be removed with the patient in his bed. Removal of a nasal pack is uncomfortable and may be painful, and the patient will be anxious. Epistaxis and epiphora can occur when the pack is removed and occasionally the patient may faint.

Before removal of packs case notes must be checked to confirm the number of packs in each nasal cavity as there may be more than one. Tilley's nasal forceps is normally the instrument of choice for removing packs.

NURSING MANAGEMENT

1   Explain the procedure to the patient, who should be in a comfortable upright position, well supported with pillows. Warn the patient that epiphora will occur; men in particular find this embarrassing if not explained. Ask the patient to breathe through his mouth until both packs are completely removed. Clothing should be protected.

2   Ask the patient to flex his neck slightly and position a small receiver, which the patient may hold, just under the anterior nares.

3   Grasp the end of one pack with the Tilley's forceps and gently remove it using a steady even pull in a forward, downward direction, dropping it into the receiver. If necessary, let the patient regain his composure before removing the pack from the other nasal cavity. Stubborn packs may be removed using toothed dissecting forceps as these give a better grip and allow more traction to be applied. In this situation analgesia is likely to be required.

4   If there is oozing a nasal bolster should be applied at once. Active bleeding should be treated by applying ice packs to the forehead and informing the doctor. Pressure should not be applied to Little's area following nasal surgery as it can cause deflection of a newly straightened septum. Should there be no ooze, or when oozing stops, the patient should be offered a mouth wash, the upper lip and external nose should be cleaned gently of any dried blood and a nasal bolster applied.

5   Following removal of packs the patient is asked to remain resting in bed for an hour. During this time the nurse should return to observe for any bleeding. The patient is asked not to blow his nose and to use disposable tissues to clean away any discharge.

6   The nasal cavities should be inspected to ensure that all of the packing has been removed.

Subsequent Care

Patients usually go home 1–2 days after the packs have been removed, taking with them any prescribed nasal drops and inhalation (Chapter 18). They will have some degree of nasal obstruction for about 2–3 weeks after surgery. Most people benefit from at least 10 days off work and away from crowded areas to reduce the likelihood of infection. Patients should be seen for review about 6 weeks post-operatively.

Complications

Complications of septal surgery are unusual, but include post-operative bleeding, septal haematoma, septal perforation, and 'saddling' of the nasal bridge-line.

SEPTAL HAEMATOMA

Aetiology

A septal haematoma is a collection of blood beneath the muco-perichondrium of the septum, which nearly always results from a blow on the nose, or a nasal operation such as septoplasty.

Clinical Features

The patient complains of nasal obstruction and examination reveals a soft swelling of the septum bulging into both nasal cavities.

Treatment

A large haematoma should be drained: antibiotic cover must be given to prevent secondary infection producing a *septal abscess*, which tends to cause necrosis of the septal cartilage and a saddle deformity of the nose. To promote drainage of the incised haematoma the patient should be nursed sitting up in bed, well supported with pillows. The haematoma blocks the nose and the nursing management is that for the patient with nasal obstruction due to nasal packs.

SEPTAL PERFORATION

Aetiology

A hole in the septum most commonly results from trauma; usually it is found to be the postoperative complication of an SMR, but occasionally other factors are responsible such as over-enthusiastic cauterization, chronic nose-picking, cocaine addiction ('sniffing snow'), and exposure to acid fumes in the chromium-plating industry. Less commonly there is underlying disease such as Wegener's granulomatosis, malignant midline granuloma, syphilis or tuberculosis.

Clinical Features

Frequently the patient is symptom free; occasionally crusting and minor epistaxis are a problem, and sometimes small perforations cause whistling on respiration. The perforation is usually situated in the anterior part of the septum.

Investigations

If there is doubt as to the pathology, a biopsy must be taken, and also a blood sample to check the ESR and syphilitic serology.

Treatment

Often no treatment is needed. If symptoms are troublesome and the defect is small, surgical closure may be attempted by rotating a mucosal flap. Large perforations are difficult to deal with, but removal of exposed cartilage may allow healing of the mucosal edges with relief of symptoms.

CHOANAL ATRESIA

Aetiology

Choanal atresia is a rare congenital condition in which one or both choanal openings fail to perforate during development of the nose—one or both nasal cavities are thus obstructed by a posteriorly situated wall of bone (or sometimes a membrane of soft tissue).

Clinical Features

Bilateral choanal atresia is a life-threatening condition—respiratory distress develops in the neonatal period due to interference with the normal pattern of obligatory nasal respiration, with inability to breathe during feeding. Unilateral choanal atresia often goes unnoticed until later life.

Investigations

The diagnosis is confirmed by failure to pass a soft rubber catheter through the nose into the pharynx; and by X-ray studies with contrast medium in the nose, or a CT scan.

Treatment

In the neonate with bilateral atresia an oral airway must be taped in place as a temporary measure. Operative treatment is urgent, and consists of drilling away the atretic plate by either a transnasal or transpalatal approach. The openings are kept open with Portex tubes for the first 6 weeks. In unilateral cases the technique is similar, but surgery may be delayed.

The newborn infant is likely to require nursing in an incubator after this operation, usually in a Special Care Baby Unit.

It is essential that regular suction is performed to keep the Portex tubes patent. If mucus begins to crust inside the tubes it can be softened with a small amount (0.25–0.5 ml) of sterile saline prior to suction. Mucus, and in the immediate postoperative period sero-sanguinous fluid, may collect around the portion of the tube that is in the nasal vestibule and this will also need to be removed by gentle suction or sterile cotton wool dressed sticks. Drainage of mucus, and secretions, can be aided by nursing the baby on alternate sides.

As his condition improves the baby can start to have breast or bottle feeds and the intravenous infusion is removed. Until oral feeding is well established, regular oral hygiene is important irrespective of the surgical approach.

It is essential that parents are kept well informed about their child's progress and that they are involved in the care of their child whenever possible.

16 Epistaxis

Epistaxis (nasal bleeding) is common; the bleeding is usually minor, but it can be severe and may be life-threatening.

AETIOLOGY

Local Causes

1 Traumatic: injury (with or without a fracture), foreign body, nose picking, nasal surgery.
2 Infective: infective rhinitis, sinusitis.
3 Neoplastic: benign or malignant tumours of the nose, sinuses or nasopharynx.
4 Idiopathic: spontaneous bleeding from dilated vessels in or near Little's area.

General Causes

1 Congenital: hereditary haemorrhagic telangiectasia.
2 Neoplastic: leukaemia.
3 Vascular: raised arterial pressure—hypertension, excitement; raised venous pressure—cardiac failure, severe cough (e.g. pneumonia).
4 Drug-induced: anticoagulants, cytotoxics.

The Commonest Causes

Of the many causes of nose bleeding, two stand out as being by far the commonest: idiopathic epistaxis and hypertensive epistaxis.

Idiopathic epistaxis is most common in children, teenagers and young adults. The bleeding arises from Little's area or nearby, is often associated with slight trauma or infection (e.g. a cold), is usually easily stopped, and tends to recur.

Hypertensive epistaxis occurs in patients who are middle aged or elderly. The bleeding tends to arise far back in the nose, and is often difficult to stop, but only sometimes recurs. It is in this group of patients that epistaxis is most dangerous.

CLINICAL FEATURES

The patient may present with the complaint of recurrent episodes of spontaneous epistaxis, and attend the clinic between bleeds. Examination almost always reveals the cause to be a leash of dilated vessels in, or near, Little's area.

Alternatively the patient may attend as an emergency with active bleeding that will not stop. Usually the bleeding is from one nostril, but it may flow back into the nasopharynx and then appear in the opposite nostril; blood may also be swallowed, in which case the amount of blood lost is not at all obvious, until it is vomited back or there is subsequent melaena. Often the bleeding point is far back and impossible to identify.

TREATMENT

The patient with recurrent spontaneous epistaxis from Little's area is effectively treated by cauterization of the offending blood vessels under local anaesthesia. The nose is first sprayed with a mixture of cocaine 10% and adrenaline 1:1000, and a pledget of cotton wool soaked in the same solution is then left in contact with the area for 10 minutes. Having removed the swab, the vessel stands out clearly and is cauterized by touching the area with either a silver nitrate stick, or with the galvano-cautery at dull red heat (many patients find this latter method alarming).

A patient coming to hospital with active epistaxis is naturally frightened and anxious even if he is aware of the cause. A sympathetic and calm approach by the nurse can do much to relieve the patient's anxiety and it is essential to give adequate explanations of the various steps in the treatment.

Vital signs are taken and recorded. It is unnecessary to obtain other than essential administrative details until the bleeding is controlled and the patient at ease (unless there is sufficient staff and someone with the patient who can give the information required). The nurse should concentrate on caring for the patient and assisting the doctor.

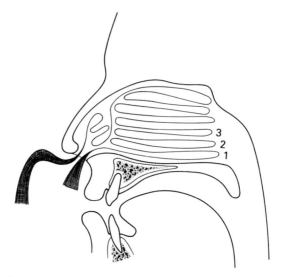

Fig. 16.1 Insertion of an anterior nasal pack. (Adapted by kind permission of Foxen E. H. M. *Lecture Notes on Diseases of the Ear, Nose and Throat*, 5th edn., p. 97. Blackwell Scientific Publications, Oxford.)

In the patient with persistent epistaxis the first priority is to stop the bleeding, using the methods outlined below.

Pressure

Pressure may suffice: the patient compresses the nostrils against the septum between finger and thumb, thus controlling bleeding from Little's area. Pressure is maintained for 10 minutes while the patient sits upright with the head flexed slightly forward, breathing through the open mouth, and spitting out any blood in the pharynx into a bowl. An ice-pack applied to the bridge of the nose is said to produce reflex vasoconstriction, and may be helpful.

Anterior Nasal Packing

Anterior nasal packing is the next step if pressure fails. Suction must be to hand. The nasal cavity which is bleeding is sprayed with a mixture of cocaine 10% and adrenaline 1:1000, and is then packed with 2.5 cm ribbon gauze wrung out in the same solution. After about 30 minutes the pack is gently removed; if there is no bleeding it may be possible to identify and cauterize the source. If bleeding re-commences, then local anaesthesia will have been

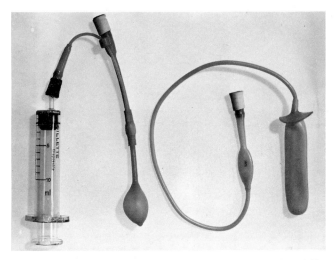

Fig. 16.2 A Brighton epistaxis balloon (left, attached to syringe) and Simpson's Bag (right).

achieved and a firm anterior nasal pack of 2.5 cm ribbon gauze soaked in vaseline or liquid paraffin can be inserted with minimum discomfort (Fig. 16.1). Alternatively, an inflatable rubber tampon (Simpson's bag or Brighton balloon) may be employed (Fig. 16.2).

A patient with an anterior nasal pack requires hospital admission, and should be nursed propped-up in bed with sufficient sedation to make him drowsy. Systemic antibiotic cover should be given if it proves necessary to leave the pack in place for more than 24 hours. A blood sample should be taken for a full blood count (including haematocrit and ESR) and for blood grouping with saved serum in case transfusion is needed.

If possible the patient's bed should be visible from the main nursing desk, but in a quiet area. Nursing management is that outlined in Chapter 15 for a patient with nasal packs *in situ* with the following additions. If a fluid balance chart is indicated it should be maintained until the packs have been out for 24 hours with no further bleeding. Bed rest is maintained for several hours after removal of the packs and nursing measures to prevent the complications of immobility must be undertaken, especially in the elderly—a physiotherapist can be of much help. Constipation results in straining and the rise in venous pressure can cause

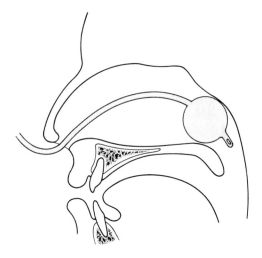

Fig. 16.3 A Foley catheter used as a post-nasal pack.

another epistaxis. Sedatives are prescribed in order to reduce anxiety and promote rest.

Post-nasal Packing

Post-nasal packing may be necessary if the bleeding is arising very far back, and bleeding continues into the nasopharynx despite anterior nasal packing. Usually a Foley catheter (or Brighton balloon) is sufficient (Fig. 16.3); it is introduced via the nostril on the side of bleeding, and the balloon is inflated with air in the post-nasal space. Gentle traction is then applied to draw the balloon against the choana, and the catheter is taped in position to the side of the face. A firm anterior nasal pack can then be inserted, and packed posteriorly against the balloon without any danger of it being swallowed.

If a Foley fails then a gauze post-nasal pack must be inserted under general anaesthesia (Fig. 16.4). The pack comprises a walnut-sized gauze plug, which is held in place by a pair of tapes led forward through each nasal cavity and tied over a dental roll across the columella; a linen thread attached to the pack and led out through the mouth facilitates removal on the ward after 24 hours. Antibiotic cover is essential for any patient with a post-nasal pack, to prevent otitis media.

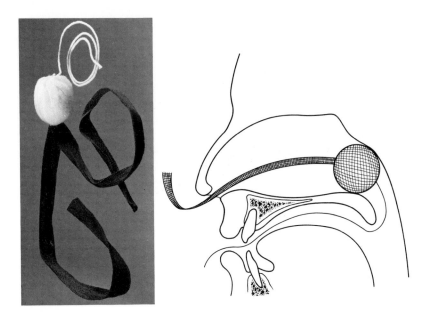

Fig. 16.4 A gauze post-nasal pack; diagram of the pack in place.

Once patients are fully recovered from the effects of the general anaesthetic they are nursed sitting up to facilitate drainage, reduce any venous congestion and promote comfort. The packs can cause a significant amount of airway obstruction. An elderly person or anyone with inadequate cardiac or pulmonary function is likely to require oxygen therapy.

It is only possible to breathe through the mouth, so regular thorough oral hygiene is essential. The dental roll in front of the columella will need to be changed at least daily to prevent excoriation of the underlying skin. The linen thread coming out of the mouth can cut the corner of the lip; generous applications of yellow soft paraffin to the area can help prevent this. This thread must always be visible and it is attached to the cheek by adhesive tape.

If the ties in front of the columella become undone the pack can slip down in the pharynx and cause respiratory obstruction. Should this occur the pack must be removed immediately by pulling on the linen thread coming out of the mouth.

A post-nasal pack is normally removed by a doctor, cutting the tapes in front of the columella and removing the pack through the mouth with the aid of the linen thread and a pair of forceps.

Fluid balance records are maintained. The pack is large, uncomfortable and prevents complete closure of the nasopharynx by the soft palate. It is unlikely that the patient is going to manage more than a fluid diet.

The pack can cause a degree of airway obstruction resulting in hypoxia and hypercarbia so observations for these need to be made. This is of particular importance in a person suffering from respiratory or cardiac disease.

Bed rest is maintained for several hours after removal of the pack. Until full mobility is reached nursing measures are undertaken to prevent the side-effects of prolonged bed rest and constipation.

The smallest amount of blood looks like a large volume to the person who is losing it and a major part of the nurse's role is to help reduce the fear and allay the anxiety suffered, by gentle reassurance and careful explanation.

Arterial Ligation

Arterial ligation is occasionally required if all the various measures detailed above fail to control the bleeding, and there is no evidence of a coagulation disorder.

If the bleeding is arising posteriorly or low down in the nasal cavity, the internal maxillary artery is ligated in the pterygopalatine fossa. A Caldwell–Luc approach (see Chapter 18) is used; the anterior, and then the posterior bony antral walls are removed to expose the artery, which is occluded with silver clips. If even this fails to stop the haemorrhage, then the external carotid artery must be ligated in the neck.

If the bleeding is arising anteriorly or high up in the nasal cavity, the anterior ethmoidal artery is clipped in the orbit, via an incision just in front of the medial canthus.

INVESTIGATION

Once the bleeding has stopped, every effort must be made to identify the cause. Sinus X-rays should be delayed for at least 2 weeks however, or else the appearances will be confused by the presence of blood in the sinuses.

17 Rhinitis and Nasal Polyps

RHINITIS

Rhinitis is a condition characterized by a triad of symptoms, any two of which may be sufficient to make the diagnosis, these are: nasal obstruction, watery rhinorrhoea and sneezing.

Aetiology

The symptoms of rhinitis are produced by an inflammatory reaction within the mucous membrane of the nose, and this reaction may be produced by various mechanisms, allergic and otherwise. The result is firstly swelling of the mucosa, due to vascular dilatation and to increased capillary permeability leading to oedema; and secondly a copious clear, watery nasal secretion due to an enormous increase in the activity of the seromucinous glands.

The various types of rhinitis are classified diagrammatically in Table 17.1. It will be noted that the term 'intrinsic rhinitis' is employed instead of the more commonly used expression 'vasomotor rhinitis'; this is because *all* types of rhinitis involve a vasomotor change in the mucosa, and it is therefore meaningless to apply the term to any one type.

Symptoms

The patient complains of nasal obstruction, which tends to fluctuate in severity and alternate from side to side, together with a watery nasal discharge (and sometimes a postnasal drip), and bouts of sneezing. In hayfever there may be an associated conjunctivitis, with itching, watering eyes.

A careful history will usually identify the cause of an extrinsic rhinitis. If the symptoms are confined to the grass pollen season,

147

Table 17.1   A classification of rhinitis.

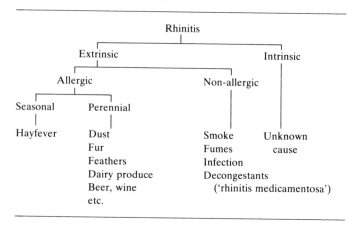

then hayfever is clearly the problem. If symptoms persist throughout the year and are exacerbated by exposure to dust, then sensitivity to dust (or the dust mite, *Dermatophagoides pteronyssinus*) is likely. Sometimes it transpires that the patient has been using nasal decongestants (vasoconstrictor preparations such as Otrivine, Sinex or Fenox) on a long-term basis, and has developed a rhinitis medicamentosa. This condition develops because the initial vasoconstrictor effect of such preparations is followed by a rebound phenomenon of vasodilatation and nasal obstruction, which the patient interprets as the signal for another dose; a vicious circle then develops, because in time the phase of vasoconstriction becomes steadily shorter and so the patient resorts to the decongestant more and more frequently.

Often the patient's symptoms are perennial with no aggravating factors, and he falls into the category of intrinsic rhinitis.

Signs

Examination reveals nasal obstruction due to enlarged turbinates and a swollen 'boggy' mucous membrane. The colour of the mucous membrane is variable; often it is unusually pale and lilac-coloured, and occasionally it is bright red, especially in cases of rhinitis medicamentosa. There may be associated nasal polyps or a co-existing septal deviation.

Investigations

Sinus X-rays should usually be performed in case there is a sinusitis; in the absence of infection, mucosal thickening in the maxillary antra is nevertheless often seen in patients with rhinitis. Skin-testing with various allergens may be helpful in confirming a diagnosis made on the basis of the history, but it must be remembered that skin sensitivity and nasal sensitivity are not necessarily the same, and misleading false-positive and false-negative results can occur.

Skin Testing

This procedure is often performed by a member of the nursing staff in the OPD. After taking a careful history to establish likely allergens, skin testing is performed to establish whether the patient is allergic to these substances, and to what extent. Antihistamine drugs should have been discontinued for 48 hours before the test is performed, as these can suppress the skin reaction. A tourniquet to prevent further spread of the testing solution through the body and injections of antihistamine and adrenaline should be at hand in case of an anaphylactic reaction. The flexor aspect of the forearm is the site most commonly used for the test. If it is necessary to clean the skin, soap and water should be used. The patient may be allergic to the solution in which the test allergens are dissolved so a control is always carried out using the solution alone. The skin can be marked with a ballpoint pen to identify the sites of the different allergens and of the control. There are three methods of skin testing.

SCRATCH TEST

The scratch test involves making a scratch on the skin, without drawing blood. A drop of the testing solution is then applied to the scratch.

PRICK-TEST

The prick test is performed by first placing a drop of the testing solution on the skin and then pricking the superficial layers of the skin with the tip of a needle through the drop of solution, without drawing blood. A fresh needle is used for each test solution. The same concentration of allergen can be used for scratch or prick test.

INTRADERMAL TEST

When intradermal testing is performed a small amount of a very much weaker testing solution is injected into the skin.

The test sites are examined about 10–15 minutes after testing for reaction. A reaction is shown by erythema and weal formation. The strength of any reaction is gauged by the degree of erythema and the size of the weal. A reaction gauge can be used to measure the size of the reaction.

Medical Treatment

Most patients with rhinitis (especially hayfever) have mild symptoms, and are effectively managed by their GP with antihistamines taken occasionally as required. Patients with severe symptoms tend to be referred for an ENT opinion, and their treatment is discussed below.

Hayfever

Clearly avoidance of places where the pollen count is likely to be high is a basic precaution. Desensitization by means of pre-seasonal injections of pollen extract is effective in some individuals; those patients who are not helped in this way are effectively treated by intranasal beclomethasone (Beconase), or sodium cromoglycate (Rynacrom) used prophylactically.

Perennial Allergic Rhinitis

Elimination of the responsible allergen can often be achieved by, for example, undertaking measures to suppress dust, by avoiding cats, dogs or other offending animals, or by adhering to a milk-free diet if dairy products are to blame. It is usually necessary however, to supplement these measures with intranasal cromoglycate or beclomethasone, or in severe cases with betamethasone (Betnesol) drops.

Non-allergic Extrinsic Rhinitis

Responsible irritants such as cigarette smoke or fumes must be avoided if at all possible, and any infective element must be treated with an appropriate antibiotic. Residual symptoms are usually controlled by intranasal beclomethasone or betamethasone drops. The treatment of rhinitis medicamentosa is to stop using the vasoconstrictor preparation responsible; the patient's symptoms become worse before becoming better, and betamethasone drops are useful to help patients over this difficult withdrawal period.

Intrinsic Rhinitis

No cause can be identified in this group, and so treatment must be symptomatic with beclomethasone, or betamethasone drops.

Surgical Treatment

Occasionally patients with a severe rhinitis fail to respond to medical treatment, and those in whom nasal obstruction is the predominant symptom can be helped by surgically reducing the size of the inferior turbinates, either by sub-mucous diathermy (SMD) or by trimming off redundant tissue.

The pre- and postoperative care can be planned from that described in Chapter 15 for surgical treatment of nasal obstruction.

Atrophic Rhinitis

Atrophic rhinitis is an ill-understood condition, fortunately rare in Britain, in which the nasal mucosa undergoes atrophy, and the nasal cavities become filled with foul-smelling crusts. A similar situation can arise following nasal operations in which one nasal cavity is greatly enlarged, for example following a lateral rhinotomy where much of the lateral wall of the nose is removed.

Treatment

Treatment with saline douches on a regular twice-daily basis helps to keep the nose free of crusts. Various forms of surgical treatment have been devised, but none is entirely satisfactory.

NASAL SNIFFS OR DOUCHE
Nasal sniffs are prescribed two or three times daily to loosen crusts or remove excess secretions from the nose. Solutions used include saline (1 teaspoon common salt in a tumblerful of warm water)

or an alkaline nasal douche (equal parts of sodium bicarbonate, sodium chloride and borax dissolved in water at body temperature). The procedure is explained to the patient and he is sat upright with his clothing protected and with privacy ensured. A disposable cup is filled to the brim with the prepared solution and handed with a receiver to the patient. The patient is asked to sniff the solution up one nostril at a time whilst compressing the other nostril with a finger. The solution is sniffed through the nasal cavity into the nasopharynx, then spat out of the mouth into the receiver. It may be necessary to top up the solution in the cup before the second side is treated, or for convenience 2 cups of solution can be given at the start. Instead of sniffing the fluid from the cup a little can be poured into the palm of one hand and the fluid sniffed from the cupped palm.

On completion the patient will appreciate some tissues to use for blowing away any excess fluid from the nose. As this procedure may result in foul tasting secretions passing through the mouth it should always be followed by brushing the teeth and gums and a pleasant tasting mouth wash.

NASAL POLYPS

Nasal polyps represent areas of nasal mucous membrane which have become oedematous, distended with intercellular fluid, and have then been pulled down by gravity as globular swellings.

Aetiology

Occasionally nasal polyps develop in association with an allergic rhinitis, but more often the rhinitis is of intrinsic type. Chronic sinusitis used to be an important cause of nasal polyposis, but it is now becoming steadily less common.

Symptoms

The predominant symptoms in nasal polyposis are nasal obstruction and anosmia: occasionally there is rhinorrhoea and sneezing as well.

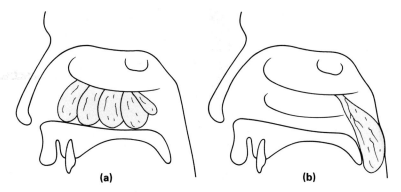

Fig. 17.1 Nasal polyps: (a) ethmoidal; (b) antrochoanal. (Adapted by kind permission from Foxen E. H. M. (1980) *Lecture Notes on Diseases of the Ear, Nose and Throat*, 5th edn., p. 130. Blackwell Scientific Publications, Oxford.

Signs

Examination reveals pale, pearly-grey globular swellings obstructing the nasal cavities, usually arising from the ethmoid region in
the middle meatus on both sides (Fig. 17.1). Malignancy is
suspected if a polyp is unilateral, ulcerated, pink and fleshy in
appearance, or if it bleeds.

Investigations

Sinus X-rays usually just show mucosal thickening in the antra, but
occasionally there is definite radiological evidence of associated
maxillary sinusitis. The ethmoid cells are generally opaque.

Medical Treatment

Mild polyposis with only a minor degree of nasal obstruction can
be successfully treated along the lines already discussed for
rhinitis. Betamethasone drops are especially useful.

Surgical Treatment

Intranasal Polypectomy

Intranasal polypectomy, using a snare and punch forceps, is usually
adequate. Unless there are only one or two polyps it is a procedure

best carried out under general anaesthesia. If concurrent maxillary sinusitis is suspected, then antral washout may be performed at the same time.

Many of these patients suffer from asthma, and may be taking steroids; this information should be obtained when the nursing history is taken. Such a patient would be nursed as near as possible to the main nursing desk and the frequency and nature of observation adjusted accordingly.

Various types and sizes of anterior nasal packs are used. They are generally removed after 12–24 hours. Care is aimed at relieving the nursing problems caused by the packs (Chapter 15) and watching for haemorrhage. The stay in hospital is short, and the patient is usually able to return to normal living patterns within 2 weeks.

Ethmoidectomy

Exenteration of the ethmoid cells may be recommended for patients with nasal polyps which recur rapidly, the principle of the procedure being to remove the roots of the polyps within the ethmoid cells. The operation may be performed either *intra-nasally*, *externally* via an incision close to the medial canthus of the eye, or *transantrally* via a Caldwell–Luc approach.

Prognosis

However thoroughly nasal polyps are removed, they tend to recur.

Antrochoanal Polyps

An antrochoanal polyp is one which arises within the maxillary antrum, extrudes through the ostium into the nose, and enlarges until it passes back through the choana into the post-nasal space (Fig. 17.1). It is a solitary polyp.

Incidence

Antrochoanal polyps are commonest in teenagers, and are much commoner in boys than girls.

Symptoms and Signs

The patient complains of unilateral nasal obstruction. Anterior
rhinoscopy, however, may reveal no abnormality, and it is only on
examination of the post-nasal space with a mirror that the polyp is
seen.

Investigations

Sinus X-rays invariably reveal opacity of the maxillary sinus on the
affected side, and the polyp is seen in the nasopharynx on the
lateral view.

Treatment

The polyp may be avulsed under general anaesthesia, by passing a
snare around the narrow pedicle where it emerges from the sinus
ostium. About half the polyps so removed will recur, however, and
in these cases it is necessary to carry out a Caldwell–Luc operation
in order to exenterate the origin of the polyp by stripping out the
antral lining. The nursing care required is described in Chapter 18.

18 Sinusitis

ACUTE SINUSITIS

Acute Maxillary Sinusitis

An acute inflammation of the mucosa of the maxillary sinus, with pain and free mucopus within the sinus.

Aetiology

Maxillary sinusitis usually develops as a result of spread of an adjacent infection (e.g. coryza or a dental infection), or from infection introduced by swimming.

Less commonly other factors predispose, such as trauma, a neoplasm in the sinus, allergic rhinitis, or the presence of a foreign body or deviated nasal septum.

Pathology

Often the initial infection is viral, and secondary bacterial infection then develops. The infection first stimulates increased mucus production from the inflamed mucosal lining of the antrum, and mucopus forms; as the infection progresses, however, the mucosa becomes necrotic, oedema and fibrin close the ostium, and the sinus becomes filled with pus. As the pressure of pus within the sinus increases pain develops, and eventually thrombophlebitis may result in spread of infection to other tissues.

Symptoms

The usual history is of a cold that becomes steadily worse, with nasal obstruction, purulent rhinorrhoea and post-nasal drip, cheek pain, a poor sense of smell and occasionally minor epistaxis.

Signs

The patient is often pyrexial, with a poor nasal airway, inflamed mucosa, and pus in the nasal cavities and post-nasal space. The sinus affected is tender to palpation.

Investigations

A nasal swab should be sent for culture and sensitivity. The tip of the swab should be passed back along the floor of the nose collecting as much pus and mucus as is possible. (When taking a nasal swab for the detection of Staphylococcus carriers it is sufficient to insert the tip of the swab into the vestibule.) Sinus X-rays show opacity of the antrum, and sometimes a fluid level (Fig. 18.1).

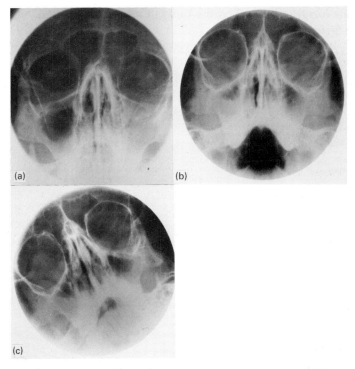

Fig. 18.1   (a) Maxillary sinusitis: opacity of the left antrum; (b) maxillary sinusitis: a fluid level in the right antrum; (c) maxillary sinusitis: fluid level confirmed by tilted view.

Treatment

Generally, acute sinusitis resolves with medical treatment, while chronic sinusitis requires surgical management.

Treatment comprises rest, plentiful oral fluids, and analgesics (e.g. paracetamol), observing for complications and recording vital signs. Specific treatment consists of an appropriate antibiotic (e.g. co-trimoxazole or amoxycillin), together with nasal decongestants (e.g. Sudafed plus 1% ephedrine nose drops and steam inhalations), given for a period of 10–14 days.

INSTILLATION OF NASAL DROPS

The patient is first asked to gently blow his nose. He is positioned supine on a bed or couch with one pillow under his shoulders and his head over the edge (Fig. 18.2).

The patient is then asked to close his eyes whilst the drops are being instilled and to breathe through his mouth during, and for the 4–5 minutes that he remains in the supine position after instillation. While the drops are being instilled into one nostril the other is compressed with a finger. If there is any likelihood of the patient moving during the procedure it is wise to protect his eyes with a gauze swab or tissue.

On completion of the treatment the patient is handed a tissue to collect any fluid from his nose which may appear when he is helped back into an upright position.

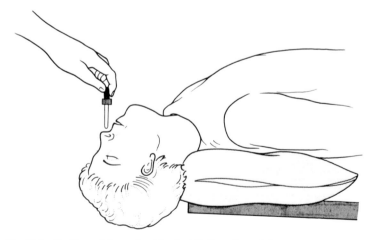

Fig. 18.2   Position of the patient for installation of nasal drops.

OPEN STEAM INHALATIONS

Open steam inhalations relieve congestion and loosen crusting in the nasal cavities. Most of the benefits of this treatment come from the effect of the steam but other substances (e.g. pine or Karvol) may be added to give a pleasant aroma. Inhalations are normally given two or three times daily immediately after decongestant drops have been used. Many patients find inhalations soothing particularly when given early in the morning and late in the evening.

In order to gain maximum benefit from the inhalation and maintain safety, the patient should be sitting upright. Spillage of the hot fluid is a potential hazard and the patient must be well protected with a waterproof drape covering shoulders, chest and lap. This should then be covered by some form of absorbent towelling.

The nurse who gives the inhalation is responsible for seeing that the patient comes to no harm. Children, the elderly and very ill or confused patients must never be left alone with an inhalation. Indeed, if risks are present, the need for inhalation should be questioned. The Nelson's inhaler (or alternatively a 1 litre jug) is placed in a bowl and surrounded by some form of packing (e.g. dressing towels) to stabilize it. This should then be placed in front of the patient on a steady table, of suitable height with the air inlet turned away from the patient. Some hospital bed tables do not fit this description and care has to be taken.

A temperature of not less than 60°C is required to vapourize an inhalant such as Karvol; the temperature at the start of the inhalation should be 70–75° to allow for cooling. This temperature can be achieved by filling a Nelson's inhaler with boiling water and leaving it to stand for 15 minutes. Alternatively by using the following quantities the correct temperature can be achieved and the level of water will not come above the air inlet:

Large Nelson's inhaler: 600 ml boiling water plus 200 ml cold tap water.

Small Nelson's Inhaler: 300 ml boiling water plus 150 ml cold tap water.

Before starting the inhalation the patient should gently blow his nose (except in the immediate postoperative period), blowing each nostril separately to clear away any loose mucus or debris. To allow the patient to be observed closely and to prevent steam coming into contact with all of the face and hair a towel can be folded into a tubular shape and one end placed around the steam outlet of the inhaler, or jug, the other end being fitted around the nose and mouth. Alternatively, a towel can be placed over the patient's head and the inhaler. The patient is asked to breathe through his nose as much as possible.

The inhalation is continued until steam is no longer present: this takes between 10–15 minutes. On completion of the inhalation the face needs to be dried and if necessary the hair combed.

ANTRAL WASHOUT

Antral washout should be avoided for the first 24 hours of treatment because of the risk of spreading infection, but it may be necessary if symptoms are unimproved and pain persists after 48 hours.

An antral washout can generally be carried out in adults under local anaesthesia. The nasal cavity is sprayed with a mixture of equal parts of 10% cocaine and 1:1000 adrenaline. Anaesthesia is completed by inserting a silver cocainising wire carrying the same solution, or 25% cocaine paste, on a cotton wool pledget beneath the inferior turbinate, and leaving it in place for 10 minutes.

The cocainising wire is then removed, and a Tilley–Lichtwitz trocar and cannula (Fig. 18.3) is inserted under the inferior turbinate with its tip as high as possible. Then, with a slight rotary motion, the instrument is pushed through the thin medial wall of the antrum, 'aiming' at the top of the pinna (Fig. 18.4). The trocar is removed, and an empty syringe is used to aspirate through the

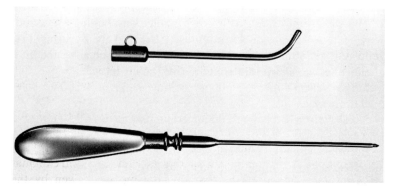

Fig. 18.3 Tilley-Lichtwitz trocar and cannula (below), and Rose's cannula (above).

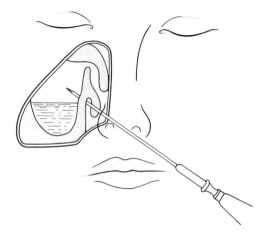

Fig. 18.4 The position of the trocar and cannula in performing an antral washout. (Adapted by kind permission from Foxen E. H. M. (1980) *Lecture Notes on Diseases of the Ear, Nose and Throat*, 5th edn., p. 111. Blackwell Scientific Publications, Oxford.

cannula in order to obtain an undiluted specimen of pus for bacteriology.

The patient is next instructed to bend forward, and to breathe only through the open mouth. The antrum is then irrigated with sterile normal saline using a Higginson's syringe connected to the cannula; the effluent emerging via the sinus ostium into the nose is collected in a receiver.

It is important to guard against incorrect placement of the cannula, as the orbit or soft tissues of the cheek can be entered, with resultant swelling at these sites when saline is injected.

NURSES ROLE IN ANTRAL WASHOUT

Following the application of cocaine the patient must be observed for toxic reaction to the drug (see Chapter 28). Should this occur the cocainising wires must be removed immediately and the medical staff informed. The patient may also feel faint from being very anxious about the procedure. Dentures should be removed to a labelled container once the cocaine has been applied, until the procedure has been completed. During this time a second explanation of the procedure (the first one having been given by the doctor) can be given and any questions that the patient may have can be answered. The correct temperature of the normal saline is

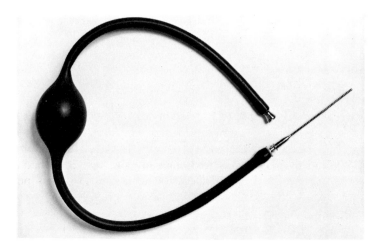

Fig. 18.5   Higginson syringe for antral irrigation, connected to a Tilley-Lichtwitz cannula.

38°C. Before the Higginson's syringe (Fig. 18.5) is connected to the cannula it is filled and all air expelled.

During the irrigation it is necessary to keep the end of the Higginson's syringe under the level of the saline. A Higginson's syringe has a one-way valve which prevents the effluent returning into the syringe and the saline, but if the end is exposed, air will be drawn into the syringe and the patient will be at risk from air embolism. Observe the cheek and orbit for swelling. Antral washout can be a rather unpleasant procedure and the patient will require appropriate support.

On completion the cannula is removed and the patient is helped to gently blow his nose to remove any remaining fluid or secretions. He is then allowed to rest until he has recovered.

If the procedure is being done in the OPD ensure that the patient has information relevant to date and time of the next appointment and medications to be used (e.g. nasal drops or steam inhalations) before he leaves the department. Directions towards the nearest tea source are often welcome at this point. Recording the procedure and labelling specimens are often included within the nurses' role.

INTRANASAL ANTROSTOMY
In patients who suffer from recurrent attacks of acute maxillary sinusitis, or in whom an acute attack fails to resolve after a full

course of antibiotics and several antral washouts, it is advisable to proceed to the next stage in treatment and perform an intranasal antrostomy.

Intranasal antrostomy is carried out under general anaesthesia. The care and preparation of the patient is outlined in Chapter 15. An opening, approximately 1.5 cm long and 1 cm high, is fashioned in the medial wall of the antrum beneath the inferior turbinate in order to provide more adequate drainage of the sinus than that afforded by the natural ostium (Fig. 18.6). If anterior nasal packs have been inserted, the nursing care described in Chapter 15 will be needed. Occasionally antral lavage is performed on a patient with an existing antrostomy—in this circumstance a Rose's cannula is used instead of a Tilley–Lichtwitz trocar and cannula, and no local anaesthesia is required. A nurse may carry out this procedure.

Ethmoiditis

The ethmoid cells are always involved in an acute sinusitis, tending to produce retro-orbital pain and contributing to the nasal obstruction and poor sense of smell. Ethmoiditis may occur in isolation in children, where it presents as oedema at the medial canthus.

Treatment

Treatment comprises the measures already described for maxillary sinusitis.

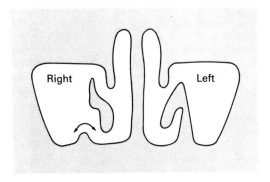

Fig. 18.6 The site for a right intranasal antrostomy. (Adapted by kind permission from Foxen E. H. M. (1980) *Lecture Notes and Diseases of the Ear, Nose and Throat*, 5th edn., p. 112. Blackwell Scientific Publications, Oxford.)

Frontal Sinusitis

Frontal sinusitis often follows swimming or flying with a cold, due to infected material being forced up the frontonasal duct under pressure. The infection is usually unilateral, producing a frontal headache which tends to be worse in the mornings and on stooping down. The floor of the sinus is tender on palpation.

Treatment

Treatment consists of the standard measures already discussed for maxillary sinusitis, together with the use of topical adrenaline under the middle turbinate to encourage drainage down the frontonasal duct. There is often a concurrent maxillary sinusitis on the same side, and if symptoms do not settle after 48 hours antral washout may speed resolution. In fulminant cases, with increasing oedema of the upper eyelid indicating imminent orbital cellulitis, the frontal sinus must be drained by making a small trephine

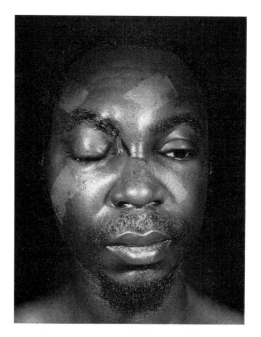

Fig. 18.7   The drain in place following trephine of the right frontal sinus.

opening through its floor via an incision beneath the medial part of the eyebrow (Fig. 18.7).

The facial wound is observed for haemorrhage and infection. As the sinus will be draining into the nose, frequent changes of nasal bolsters will be necessary. Regular eye care will be required until the oedema subsides.

Sphenoiditis

Sphenoiditis is difficult to diagnose in isolation; it often occurs in conjunction with ethmoiditis, producing a central headache and sometimes a purulent post-nasal drip.

Treatment

Treatment comprises the measures already described for maxillary sinusitis.

CHRONIC SINUSITIS

Chronic sinusitis involves chronic inflammation of the mucosa of the paranasal sinuses.

Aetiology

Chronic sinusitis is usually a sequel to a coryza, with sub-acute sinus infection, following which adequate drainage fails to be re-established. The presence of rhinitis, nasal polyps, or a mark-edly deviated nasal septum predisposes to chronic sinusitis, as does a low resistance to infection on the part of the patient.

Symptoms

These are similar to those of acute sinusitis, namely nasal obstruction, purulent rhinorrhoea and post-nasal drip, a poor sense of smell, and sometimes minor epistaxis—facial pain, however, is not usually a feature. Secondary effects of chronic sinusitis may be manifest in the form of pharyngitis, recurrent tonsillitis, laryngitis, secretory otitis media, or chronic suppurative otitis media.

Signs

Typically there is nasal airway obstruction, with inflamed mucosa, pus and crusting in the nasal cavities and post-nasal space, and often nasal polyps.

Investigations

Sinus X-rays show mucosal thickening; sometimes there is a fluid level, and there may be sclerosis of the bony sinus walls. Antral washout (proof puncture) confirms the presence of pus.

Treatment: Conservative Measures

Conservative measures consist of attending to the patient's general health, and treating acute exacerbations of infection along the lines already outlined for acute sinusitis, including antral washouts and the fashioning of intranasal antrostomies if need be. Predisposing factors, such as septal deviation, nasal polyps, or carious teeth should be corrected.

Treatment: Radical Surgery

Radical surgery is needed if conservative measures fail. The principle of radical surgery is to remove all diseased mucosal lining, and to create adequate drainage. The operation employed depends upon which sinus, or combination of sinuses, is affected.

Maxillary Sinus: Caldwell–Luc Operation

Where the maxillary sinus is affected, treatment is by Caldwell–Luc operation. In this procedure the anterior bony wall of the antrum is opened via an incision in the mucosa of the gingivolabial sulcus, under the upper lip (Fig. 18.8). The whole diseased lining membrane of the sinus can then be removed, and finally an intranasal antrostomy is created to provide permanent drainage.

NURSING CARE
The patient is prepared for a general anaesthetic. As there is going to be an incision under the upper lip the edentulous patient is

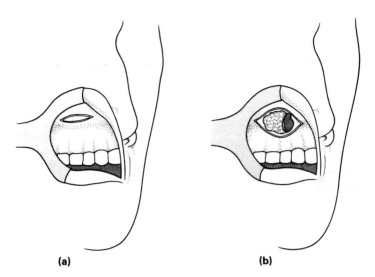

(a) **(b)**

Fig. 18.8 The Caldwell-Luc operation. (a) The sublabial incision; (b) the sublabial antrostomy, through which it can be seen that an intranasal antrostomy has been created. (Adapted by kind permission from Foxen E. H. M. (1980) *Lecture Notes on Diseases of the Ear, Nose and Throat*, 5th edn., p. 113. Blackwell Scientific Publications, Oxford.)

warned against wearing an upper denture for about a week after the operation.

After surgery the cheek on the operated side is rather swollen and ice packs may be comforting. There may also be epiphora on this side due to obstruction of the lacrimal duct so regular bathing of the eye is carried out for as long as necessary.

The surgery will result in a fair, if temporary, degree of nasal obstruction with resultant mouth breathing. Regular thorough oral hygiene with a small soft toothbrush is necessary and should be supplemented with mouthwashes of warm normal saline to keep the wound as clean and healthy as possible. This is particularly important after meals.

The sutures, if used, are of catgut and will not need to be removed. However, just as the smallest ulcer in the mouth can feel like a large crater, these sutures can cause discomfort and the tendency to keep prodding them with the tongue needs to be discouraged.

Those unable to wear dentures will benefit from a soft diet, otherwise as normal a diet as is tolerable can be taken, bearing in mind the amount of chewing necessary to eat the products of some hospital kitchens.

Some relief from nasal obstruction is obtained by the use of vasoconstricting nasal drops and steam inhalations. These are usually ordered to commence 24 hours after surgery or after the removal of any antral or nasal packs. The amount and type of analgesia required varies with the needs of each patient.

Some of the nerves to the upper teeth and gum in the area below the incision may have been damaged at the time of operation. Temporary or permanent numbness in this area may occur and prior to discharge the patient is advised to tell his dentist that this operation has been performed.

ANTRAL PACKS

To prevent bleeding following surgery the maxillary sinus may be packed with ribbon gauze impregnated with BIPP, yellow soft paraffin, or Whitehead's varnish. Alternatively a Foley's catheter may be inserted into the sinus. The balloon of the catheter should be inflated with air not water, in case it bursts whilst the patient is asleep. The catheter is brought out of the antrum via the intranasal antrostomy, through the nasal cavity and onto the face, where it is held in place with strapping. The end of the ribbon gauze pack may be left in the nasal cavity. As the pack is held in position by the walls of the sinus there is no danger of it falling into the nose and then the pharynx, so the possibility of inhalation does not exist. Anterior nasal packing may be *in situ* at the same time as the antral pack or balloon.

The nursing care of a patient with an antral pack or balloon is the same as that for a patient with an anterior nasal pack. However, the patient is likely to suffer more discomfort, pain and soft tissue swelling of the face. A cool pack applied to the swollen area can help reduce swelling; alternatively a warm pack can help relieve discomfort. Soiled strapping will need to be changed.

When anterior nasal packs are not present gentle nasal toilet using cotton wool dressed sticks soaked in warm, normal saline or sodium bicarbonate may be needed to remove mucus and debris.

REMOVAL OF THE ANTRAL PACK OR BALLOON

A doctor may prefer to remove an antral pack or balloon himself. If an anterior nasal pack is *in situ* it will need to be removed first, but not before sedation or analgesia has been given. The procedure for removal of an anterior nasal pack is described in Chapter 15. After being given an explanation the patient is helped into a comfortable upright position in bed, with his clothing protected. Warn the patient that epiphora will occur, and ask him to breathe through his mouth during removal of the catheter or pack. A receiver is held in place under the anterior nares to collect the pack or balloon.

When removing an antral balloon the strapping which is holding the catheter in place on the face is removed and the balloon is deflated using a 20 ml syringe. The end of the catheter is grasped and it is withdrawn by gently pulling downwards and towards the opposite side of the face. The catheter usually slides out very easily with a minimum of discomfort to the patient.

When removing an antral ribbon gauze pack the patient will require a truthful explanation as it is uncomfortable. A second nurse should be present to give support and reassurance. It is essential that analgesia and/or sedation is given, and allowed time to act, before the pack is removed. If the end of the pack is strapped to the face, remove the strapping. If the end is inside the nasal cavity it will be necessary to look into the patient's nose using a Thudichum nasal speculum, a source of light and a head mirror to find the end. The end of the pack is grasped with either Tilley's nasal or toothed dissecting forceps and the pack is removed as gently as possible by pulling the ribbon gauze downwards and towards the opposite side of the face. These packs can be quite stubborn and difficult to remove and it may be necessary to stop several times during removal to ease the discomfort experienced by the patient. Removal of the pack may cause some epistaxis. Should this occur, an ice pack can be applied over the cheek and nose of the affected side. After removal, check the pack to ensure that it has not been broken, leaving a portion in the sinus.

CARE FOLLOWING REMOVAL
Following removal of either a catheter or pack, a nasal bolster should be applied, and a receiver, tissues and call bell made available. The patient is asked to spit into the receiver any fluid that he can feel trickling down his throat from the nasopharynx.

The patient is then left to sit quietly in bed for about an hour or until any bleeding has subsided. During this time the nurse who performed removal should return several times to ensure that the patient is not bleeding. If blood loss is heavy then frequent observation of vital signs should be commenced, an ice pack applied and a doctor informed.

If the patient's condition is satisfactory at the end of the rest period the external nose and face can be washed clean of any dried blood, and a mouth wash offered. Advise the patient against blowing his nose for the next 24 hours. The nose can then be blown gently, one side at a time.

Ethmoid Sinuses

Treatment is by intranasal ethmoidectomy or external ethmoidectomy; fronto-ethmoidectomy (if the frontal sinus is also involved); or transantral ethmoidectomy (if the antrum is also involved).

Frontal Sinus

Treatment is generally by fronto-ethmoidectomy.

Sphenoid sinus

Treat by intranasal drainage.

Treatment: Obliterative Surgery

Obliterative surgery may be necessary if chronic frontal sinusitis fails to resolve following fronto-ethmoidectomy. Various techniques may be employed in order to obliterate the sinus so that there is simply no longer a cavity that can become infected.

COMPLICATIONS OF SINUSITIS

Sinusitis is a mucosal disease. Complications arise when infection spreads beyond the sinus walls by direct spread, by thrombophlebitis, or by embolism.

Complications are fortunately rare today, but when they do occur they usually arise from the frontal sinus in adults, and the ethmoids in children. The following complications may arise:

1   Orbital cellulitis, which may progress to cavernous sinus thrombosis.
2   Osteomyelitis of the frontal bone.

3 Intracranial complications: extradural abscess, subdural abscess, meningitis, encephalitis, cerebral abscess, sagittal sinus thrombosis and resultant hydrocephalus.

Frontal Mucocoele

Obstruction of the frontonasal duct may result in an encysted collection of mucus in the sinus, termed a mucocoele. This tends to gradually enlarge, causing frontal swelling with thinning of surrounding bone, and displacement of the eye. If a mucocoele becomes infected it is termed a pyocoele.

Treatment

Treatment consists of excision via a fronto-ethmoidectomy approach with the establishment of intranasal drainage.

19 Facial Pain

Patients who complain of pain in or around the face may be referred to an ENT surgeon, a neurologist or a dentist; for in this field there is a great deal of overlap between the specialities. Furthermore, diagnosis is complicated by the fact that referred pain is especially common in the head and neck; in this phenomenon, pain arising at one site is perceived by the patient as arising at another site subserved by a different branch of the same sensory nerve. Perhaps the commonest example of this in ENT practice is the post-tonsillectomy patient who complains of earache—examination reveals the ear to be normal, and in fact the pain is being referred from the tonsil as both the tonsil and part of the middle ear are supplied by branches of the glossopharyngeal nerve.

There is no doubt that a careful history is the most important step in identifying the cause of facial pain; although examination of the ears, nose, throat and if necessary the teeth and central nervous system, must not be neglected.

NEURAL PAIN

Nasal Neuralgias

Sinusitis

Many patients are referred to an ENT surgeon on the assumption that their headache or facial pain is due to sinusitis. This is usually not the case, for while acute sinusitis (particularly affecting the frontal sinus) is often intensely painful, chronic infection frequently does not give rise to pain.

Rhinitis

In rhinitis mucosal congestion in the nose may occlude the ostium of a sinus, resulting in pressure change within the sinus and consequent pain. The frontonasal duct is particularly liable to be affected, producing frontal headache.

Sluder's Neuralgia (Anterior Ethmoidal Syndrome)

In Sluder's Neuralgia contact between the anterior end of the middle turbinate and the nasal septum can provoke pain along the bridge of the nose, due to pressure on branches of the anterior ethmoidal nerve. If cocainisation of the middle turbinate and adjacent septum temporarily abolishes the pain, then permanent relief may be derived from an SMR, and/or out-fracture or trimming of the middle turbinate.

Septal Impaction

Occasionally a septal spur impacted against the lateral wall of the nose may give rise to facial pain, which sometimes mimics migraine. As with Sluder's neuralgia, surgical correction is only indicated if cocainisation of the area abolishes the pain.

Traumatic Neuralgia

A soft-tissue injury at the point of emergence of a branch of the trigeminal nerve may locally damage the nerve, and produce persistent pain in the area. For example, cheek pain may follow a Caldwell–Luc operation due to damage to the infra-orbital nerve, and if it persists transantral resection of the nerve may be necessary to abolish it.

Dental Neuralgias

Dental neuralgias are the commonest of all causes of facial pain. Pain usually arises from infection of the pulp space or periodontal membrane due to dental caries, or from the presence of an impacted, unerupted tooth.

Other Neuralgias

Trigeminal Neuralgia (tic doloureux)

Trigeminal neuralgia occurs in the elderly, and is of unknown cause. Brief episodes of severe, stabbing pain confined to the facial distribution area of the trigeminal nerve, and often triggered by touching the area, are characteristic and are usually abolished by carbamazepine. Pressure on the trigeminal nerve, for instance from a nasopharyngeal carcinoma, may produce a similar pain.

Glossopharyngeal Neuralgia

Glossopharyngeal neuralgia produces a similar pain to that of trigeminal neuralgia, except that the tonsillar region or ear are involved; swallowing frequently provokes the pain. Treatment with carbamazepine is less successful than in trigeminal neuralgia, and surgical treatment with section of the nerve may be required. Pressure on the nerve from, for example, an elongated styloid process may produce similar glossopharyngeal pain (relieved by excision of the offending styloid process).

Cervical Neuralgia

Cervical neuralgia may follow injuries to the cervical spine. Pain arising in the intervertebral joints and ligaments is referred via the greater occipital nerve to produce occipitofrontal headache.

Central Nervous System Lesions

Pain in the distribution of the trigeminal nerve may follow ophthalmic herpes (post-herpetic neuralgia), and may also be a feature of various brainstem lesions, notably disseminated sclerosis.

OCULAR PAIN

Less than 5% of headaches are due to disorders involving the eye. 'Eye strain' resulting from the effect of accommodation for close work, especially in long-sighted individuals, can produce local discomfort and frontal headache, and similar pain can result from acute iritis and acute glaucoma.

MUSCLE AND JOINT PAIN

Temporomandibular joint dysfunction is not uncommon. The joint becomes painful due to the stresses produced by various forms of dental malocclusion, and associated spasm of the muscles of mastication makes the discomfort worse. The pain tends to be worse on jaw movement, the joint is often tender to palpation, and it may be felt to 'click' when the mouth is opened and closed. Most cases respond readily to dental measures designed to restore normal occlusion, and a temporary prosthetic device termed a bite-raiser may be used to achieve this.

VASCULAR PAIN

Migrainous Neuralgia

Migrainous neuralgia is caused by episodic, painful distension of facial blood vessels, and produces a classical combination of symptoms which usually occurs in young men. There is intense, unilateral, throbbing facial pain centred around the eye, associated with redness and watering of the affected eye and nasal obstruction on the same side. The pain recurs regularly on a daily basis, often at about 2 am, and lasts $\frac{1}{2}$–2 hours; after a spell of some weeks there is a period of freedom before the attacks recommence (hence the old name 'cluster headaches'). Ergotamine tartrate is a highly effective treatment.

Temporal Arteritis

Temporal arteritis is an autoimmune condition in which the superficial temporal arteries become inflamed and tender, producing scalp pain and headache. Progression to involve the retinal arteries produces blindness, and immediate steroid therapy is essential.

PSYCHOGENIC PAIN

Sometimes facial pain may be of psychogenic origin, but clearly all possible organic causes must be excluded before this diagnosis is made.

PART III · THE THROAT

20 Applied Anatomy of the Mouth and Throat

THE MOUTH (Fig. 20.1)

The mouth is a cavity bounded by the cheeks, lips, hard and soft palates and the floor of the mouth (mainly the tongue). Posteriorly it is in continuity with the oropharynx at the anterior faucial pillars, the free edge of the soft palate and the posterior part of the tongue. The first teeth (the central incisors) appear at about 6–9 months old and the rest appear over the next 5 years to give a total of 20 deciduous teeth, which are shed by the age of 12 years. There are 32 teeth in the full adult complement, 8 in each half of the lower and upper jaw, appearing in sequence as the face grows, the last (wisdom teeth) coming through in late adolescence. The teeth are held in the bones by their 'roots' and the alveolar part of the bones which carry the teeth are covered with the gums (gingivae). Outside the rows of the teeth are the cheek pouches which end blindly superiorly and inferiorly at the upper and lower buccal sulci. Anteriorly these continue behind the lips as the upper and lower gingivolabial sulci. Posteriorly it is possible to insinuate a finger or instrument behind the last teeth. Via this route, access can be obtained to administer fluids when the mouth cannot be opened (e.g. after dental wiring or fracture of the jaw).

At rest, the dorsum of the tongue is in contact with the hard palate. At its edges it is in contact with the teeth and below this the surface of the tongue becomes continuous with the lingual gingivae at the gingivolingual sulci. Anteriorly the tip of the tongue is free; here it has an undersurface which lies on the anterior part of the floor of the mouth. The tongue is a mobile muscular organ attached to the hyoid bone which can be felt high in the neck behind the chin.

The ducts from the right and left parotid and the submandibular and the sublingual salivary glands open into the oral cavity. There

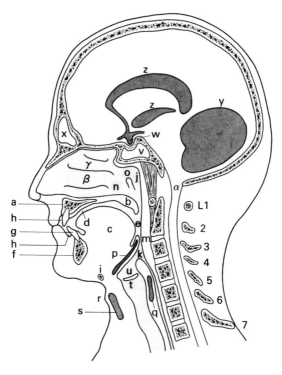

Fig. 20.1 Sagittal section through head and neck (after removal of nasal septum)—diagrammatic. (a) Hard palate; (b) soft palate; (c) tongue; (d) mouth cavity; (e) oropharynx; (f) mandible; (g) central upper and lower incisor teeth; (h) upper and lower labio-gingivol sulci; (i) hyoid bone; (j) naso pharynx; (k) laryngo pharynx; (l) 1–7 cervical vertebrae; (m) prevertebral fascia; (n) region of posterior choana; (o) Eustachian tube orifice; (p) epiglottis; (q) cricoid cartilage; (r) Adam's apple; (s) thyroid cartilage; (t) vocal cord; (u) ventricular band; (v) sphenoid sinus; (w) pituitary gland; (x) frontal sinus; (y) cerebellum; (z) representation of midline brain structures; (α) spinal canal—contains spinal cord; (β) inferior turbinate; (γ) middle turbinate.

are also numerous small mucous glands scattered beneath the mucosal aspect of the lips and cheeks.

THE PHARYNX

The pharynx can be likened to a cylinder some 10–13 cm long, divided into the nasopharynx behind the nose, the oropharynx

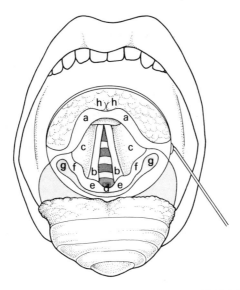

Fig. 20.2 The view obtained by indirect laryngoscopy. (a) Epiglottis; (b) vocal cord; (c) false cord; (d) interanytenoid region; (e) arytenoid cartilage; (f) aryepiglottic fold; (g) pyriform fossa; (h) vallecula. (Adapted by kind permission from Foxen E. H. M. (1980) *Lecture Notes on Diseases of the Ear, Nose and Throat*, 5th edn., p. 155. Blackwell Scientific Publications, Oxford.)

behind the mouth and the laryngopharynx behind the larynx (Fig. 20.2). Just lateral to the pharynx run the 'great vessels' of the neck—the internal jugular veins and the carotid arteries (common, internal and external). Behind lie the upper six cervical vertebrae separated from the cavity of the pharynx by a strong layer of fibrous tissue (the prevertebral fascia) to which the pharyngeal mucosa is firmly attached.

The Nasopharynx

The anterior limit of the nasopharynx is marked in the midline by the posterior end of the nasal septum and alongside this the cavity is continuous with the right and left nasal fossae via the choanae. Immediately below this hangs the mobile muscular soft palate. The roof of the nasopharynx is the base of the skull and here lie the adenoids in children. (They gradually become smaller during late childhood and have generally almost disappeared by the age of twelve). Posteriorly is the body of the first cervical vertebra. Laterally are the orifices of the lower ends of the Eustachian tubes.

The Oropharynx

The oropharynx lies in front of the second cervical vertebra. At its junction with the mouth, small muscles run down from the palate raising two folds of mucosa on each side (the anterior and posterior faucial pillars) between which lie the tonsils.

The Laryngopharynx

The laryngopharynx is in front of the third, fourth, fifth and sixth cervical vertebrae. Anteriorly is the inlet of the larynx and the epiglottis, lateral to which are the pyriform fossae which form a gutter on each side of the larynx. Below, the laryngopharynx becomes continuous with the oesophagus at the level of the cricoid cartilage. At this point the food passage is surrounded by a ring of muscle fibres forming the cricopharyngeal sphincter. This is normally closed but relaxes on swallowing to allow the passage of the food bolus.

The Larynx

The larynx is the upper continuation of the trachea and like the trachea it has a cartilaginous skeleton. The firm prominence in the front of the neck (the 'Adam's apple') is formed by the thyroid cartilage which protects the front and sides of the airway. Immediately below it is the cricoid cartilage which forms a complete ring around the airway. Within the larynx, two folds of mucosa on each side extend from the junction of the thyroid cartilages anteriorly to the cricoid cartilage posteriorly. These folds comprise the vocal cords inferiorly and the ventricular bands superiorly (also called the 'true' and 'false' cords, Fig. 20.3); between them is the opening of a blind sac called the laryngeal ventricle. The lower ends of the thyroid cartilages form a joint on each side with the cricoid cartilage which allows a very slight movement. Behind this joint is the recurrent laryngeal nerve which supplies the muscles attached to the laryngeal cartilages.

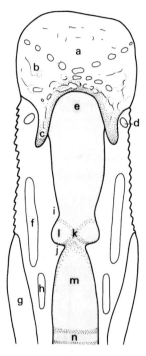

Fig. 20.3 Vertical (coronal) section through larynx, viewed from behind, diagrammatic. (a) Tongue, upper aspect; (b) tongue, posterior aspect; (c) pyriform
sinus—a gutter extending around the sides of the larynx, open posteriorly into the
food passage (pharynx); (d) hyoid bone—this gives attachment for the main
muscles of the tongue; (e) epiglottis; (f) thyroid cartilage; (g) thyroid gland;
(h) cricoid cartilage; (i) ventricular band; (j) vocal fold—the free border is the
vocal cord; (k) anterior commissure; (l) laryngeal sinus—this pocket has a variable
upward extent, in extreme cases reaching above the thyroid cartilage to form a
laryngocoele; (m) subglottis—the region surrounded by the cricoid cartilage;
(n) trachea.

The Epiglottis

The epiglottis is a plate of cartilage shaped like a leaf. It is attached
by its lower end (the stem of the leaf) to the junction of the thyroid
cartilages. From this attachment, it rises upwards behind the
tongue and its tip can sometimes be seen through the open mouth
when the tongue is pressed downwards.

21 Physiology of the Mouth and Throat

THE MOUTH

The primary task of the mouth is the preparation of food for the digestive tract. The formation of the teeth, mobility of the jaw and the mobility and covering of the tongue are adapted to the diet. Chunks of solid food are reduced by chewing which involves antero-posterior sliding and side-to-side movements of the jaws as well as opening and closing. In this process the food becomes covered with saliva, secreted by the salivary glands, and by mucus. Saliva is secreted continually during waking hours but secretion ceases during sleep. Its secretion is stimulated by food and only then does it contain digestive enzymes. The surfaces which which food comes into firm contact, that is, the palate, the dorsum of the tongue and the gingivae, are covered with tough keratinizing epithelium, firmly held to the subjacent structures. Elsewhere in the mouth the lining is not so tough (non-keratinizing). The act of swallowing is initiated voluntarily. The first stage commences with the tongue being pressed against the hard palate. The hyoid bone (and the attached larynx) is elevated, and the food pushed backwards into the oropharynx. As this happens, the soft palate is elevated, closing off the nasopharynx, and air flow through the respiratory tract is temporarily arrested.

The mouth is essential for speech. Vowel sounds are made by appropriate shaping of the mouth cavity, and consonants by appropriate movements of the tongue and lips, while vibrating air is expelled.

THE PHARYNX

In the nasopharynx and oropharynx are distributed scattered collections of lymphoid tissue. These collections are aggregated into named masses (the adenoids and the tonsils) but are often also prominent on the tongue, and the lateral and posterior walls of the pharynx.

The nasopharynx is the only part of the pharynx intended exclusively for the passage of air. Although it can be closed off from the oropharynx, it has rigid walls and cannot collapse. This contrasts with the remainder of the pharynx which is mobile and surrounded by a muscular coat, which, by contraction, propels food onwards into the oesophagus. Once food or saliva has reached the oropharynx, the remainder of the act of swallowing is reflex and involuntary. This ensures that food is in the airway for only a limited time. In this second stage of swallowing, as the larynx rises, the laryngeal inlet closes and the vocal cords come together. This protects the lower respiratory tract from inhalation of foreign material. The cricopharyngeal sphincter opens momentarily to allow food to pass into the oesophagus. Thereupon the third stage of swallowing commences and the food is propelled by peristalsis down to the stomach. The oropharynx and laryngopharynx form a passage for air and food. This region is lined by a tough mucosa which contrasts with the more delicate ciliated epithelium lining the rest of the respiratory tract as far as the smaller bronchioles. The airway will be occluded if the tongue falls backwards, for example in the unconscious patient; hence such a patient is often nursed in the coma position. This position also allows vomit or blood to escape so that it is not inhaled.

The Larynx

The essential function of the larynx is to prevent foreign material from entering the lower respiratory tract. The lining of the larynx, trachea and bronchi is very sensitive and when touched, reflex coughing occurs. In coughing the larynx is closed by the apposition (adduction) of the true and false cords and at the same time the expiratory muscles (intercostals and diaphragm) contract. This raises the pressure in the chest and when, in the next moment, the larynx opens again, there is an explosive rush of air through the bronchi, trachea and larynx which may be successful in removing the material.

The protective mechanism of the larynx depends on sensation and muscular activity, subserved by the superior and recurrent laryngeal nerves.

The phonatory function of the larynx is discussed in Chapter 25. Glottic closure allows fixation of the chest thus permitting efficient use of the shoulder muscles as in lifting.

22 Clinical Assessment of the Throat

SYMPTOMS

There are three major symptoms related to the throat.

Sore Throat

A sore throat is the commonest pharyngeal symptom. It may be severe, acute and bilateral as in tonsillitis, or it may be even more severe but unilateral as in a quinsy. A pharyngeal tumour may cause pain in the throat of gradually increasing severity. Pharyngitis, a low-grade inflammation of the pharyngeal mucosa, produces a persistent mild sore throat, which may be described by the patient as a 'dry, uncomfortable feeling'. Pain in the pharynx may be referred to the ear (see Chapter 19).

Dysphagia

Dysphagia (difficulty or discomfort on swallowing) is an alarming symptom which takes the patient quickly to his doctor. Its various causes are discussed in Chapter 25, but there are some characteristics of the type of dysphagia which give useful clues to the underlying pathology. Dysphagia which is worst for solids indicates a structural lesion causing mechanical obstruction (e.g. carcinoma of the oesophagus); dysphagia which is worst for fluids suggests a neuromuscular lesion (e.g. motor neurone disease), whereas dysphagia only when swallowing saliva makes a functional cause a strong possibility (globus pharyngeus).

Hoarseness

Hoarseness of the voice is discussed in Chapter 25. Any lesion which prevents the vocal cords meeting along their entire length will cause hoarseness, for example, inflammation (laryngitis), a tumour, or paralysis of a vocal cord.

EXAMINATION

A head mirror is used for illumination when examining the throat.

Inspection of the Throat

Inspection of the face, lips and neck is carried out first, to look for any swelling or scars, and to examine a tracheostome if one is present.

The oral cavity is next examined systematically, using two Lack tongue-depressor blades. First the teeth, alveolar margins and hard palate are inspected and then, pressing the cheeks outwards on each side with the tongue depressors, each buccal sulcus is examined, including the opening of each parotid duct. The patient is next asked to protrude his tongue, and its dorsal surface and each lateral border is examined; he is then asked to place the tip of his tongue behind the upper teeth, permitting a view of the anterior floor of the mouth. The lateral part of the floor of the mouth is then examined; again two tongue-depressors are needed to obtain a good view of this rather hidden area between the lateral border of the tongue and the lower alveolus.

The oropharynx is then examined; a Lack blade is used to depress the tongue and obtain a view of the tonsils, posterior wall of oropharynx and soft palate.

Posterior Rhinoscopy

Posterior rhinoscopy is part of the examination of the throat as well as of the nose (see Chapter 14).

Indirect Laryngoscopy

Indirect laryngoscopy is then performed. The patient is asked to open his mouth widely and protrude his tongue, which is held out gently with the aid of a piece of gauze (Fig. 22.1). He is then instructed to breathe with short panting breaths through the mouth, and a pre-warmed laryngeal mirror is introduced into the

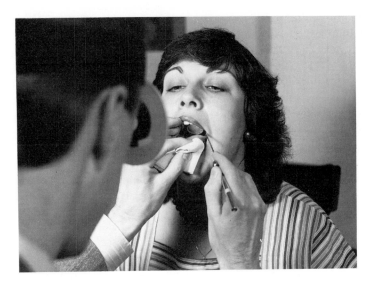

Fig. 22.1   Indirect laryngoscopy.

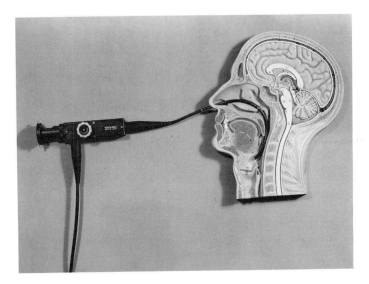

Fig. 22.2   The fibreoptic naspharyngoscope in position in an anatomical model.

mouth and pressed against the soft palate. A view is thus obtained of the base of the tongue, valleculae, epiglottis and upper part of the hypopharynx. The patient is then asked to say 'E-e-e . . .' or 'Hey . . .', and to maintain the note for as long as possible; this tips the epiglottis forward to give a view of the larynx, and allows the movements of the vocal cords to be assessed (Fig. 20.2). Some patients find it difficult to tolerate indirect laryngoscopy without gagging, and in order to obtain a view it is necessary to anaesthetize the soft palate with a lignocaine spray, or an amethocaine or benzocaine lozenge. If mirror examination is still unsuccessful, then a view may be obtained using a Hopkins rod telescope with a 90° viewing angle, or a flexible fibreoptic naso-pharyngoscope (Fig. 22.2). See also Chapter 25.

Palpation

Finally the neck is palpated, feeling for enlarged lymph nodes or other pathology.

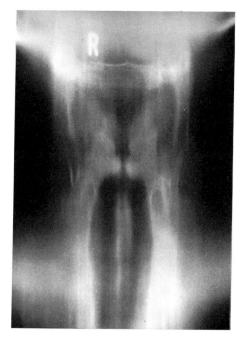

Fig. 22.3 Normal coronal tomogram of the larynx.

RADIOLOGICAL INVESTIGATIONS

Plain Lateral Soft-tissue X-ray

A plain lateral soft-tissue X-ray of the neck can provide valuable information by demonstrating soft-tissue swellings.

Tomograms

Tomograms may provide additional information (Fig. 22.3), particularly in assessing the extent of a tumour, and so may a CT scan. The old technique of laryngography, whereby a radio-opaque contrast medium was used to outline the interior of the larynx, is now seldom necessary.

A barium swallow is used to outline abnormalities of the oesophagus in the investigation of dysphagia.

23 Miscellaneous Conditions of the Mouth and Neck

CONGENITAL DEFORMITIES

Congenital deformities of the head and neck are important as they produce disfigurement and dysfunction.

Bifid uvula

Possibly the commonest congenital defect is a bifid uvula, resulting from a failure of the right and left sides of the soft palate to unite completely. This is of no significance, but a more severe degree of non-union results in *cleft palate*. In many cases the cleft extends anteriorly to involve the lip, a condition termed hare lip, which may be unilateral or bilateral. Less commonly there is a cleft of the lip with a normal palate (for treatment see Chapter 25).

Pierre Robin Syndrome

The Pierre Robin syndrome is characterized by a small lower jaw together with a cleft palate; intermittent respiratory obstruction results from inadequate mandibular support for the tongue which falls posteriorly into the pharynx.

Choanal Atresia

Choanal Atresia results from the failure of the breakdown of a partition which in early foetal life closes off the nasal cavity from the nasopharynx (see Chapter 15).

Thyroglossal Cyst

A thyroglossal cyst is a developmental abnormality in the track which the thyroid gland makes in its descent from the floor of the mouth. It is seen as a lump near the midline in the region of the hyoid bone. It is not generally very obvious in the small child because of the short neck and the bulk of the subcutaneous tissue. It is generally excised together with the central portion of the hyoid bone; if inadequately excised a *thyroglossal fistula* results.

Branchial Fistula

A branchial (cervical) fistula is a track extending from the pharynx internally to an external orifice lower in the neck.

Branchial Cyst

A branchial cyst presents as a lump, generally several centimetres in diameter, in the neck. There is not universal agreement as to whether this is a congenital developmental anomaly or not. It is of no great consequence to the patient unless it becomes infected but excision is generally advised.

NON-CONGENITAL

Lymph Nodes

The finding of enlarged lymph nodes in the neck is of the greatest clinical importance. These are enlarged in bacterial infection (e.g. of the scalp in which case one must suspect infestation with ectoparasites), in exanthemata (particularly rubella), and in glandular fever. Tuberculous lymph nodes in the neck are initially firm; if they break down a tuberculous abscess forms which may discharge on to the neck. Treatment is a combination of antituberculous chemotherapy and surgery as appropriate. Large painless nodes are a cardinal feature of Hodgkin's lymphoma—a disease predominantly affecting the young adult. Careful palpation for hard metastatic nodes in the neck is important in patients with carcinoma.

Laryngocoele (Fig. 23.1)

This is an uncommon condition in which there are pouches in communication with the airway in the larynx. These pouches may

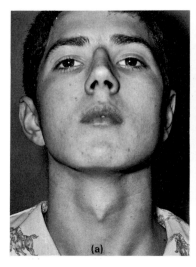
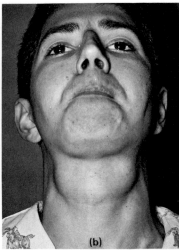

(a)   (b)

Fig. 23.1   Laryngocoele: an uncommon condition in which there are pouches in communication with the airway in the larynx. These pouches may be inflated when the patient raises the pressure in the airways: here the patient in (b) is attempting to expel air against a closed mouth and a closed nasopharynx—the inflated pouches on each side of the neck are clearly seen.

be inflated when the patient raises the pressure in the airways. Figure 23.1(b) shows the patient attempting to expel air against a closed mouth and a closed nasopharynx; the inflated pouches on each side of the neck are clearly seen.

Conditions of the Salivary Glands

Presence of a Calculus

The commonest condition of the salivary glands is the presence of a stone (calculus) in the duct of the gland which thereby becomes blocked. This results in painful enlargement of the gland behind the obstruction particularly when the gland is active (e.g. at mealtimes). The stagnation encourages secondary infection producing sialadenitis. The submandibular gland is the most commonly involved in this disease; parotid calculi are uncommon. Treatment is by removal of the stone if this is palpable in the floor of the mouth and this may be done under local anaesthetic as a straightforward outpatient procedure. Where there is recurrent trouble or where the calculus cannot be reached via the mouth, excision of the whole gland via an incision in the neck is recommended.

Pleomorphic Salivary Adenoma

Tumours of the salivary glands are commoner in the parotid. The commonest is the pleomorphic salivary adenoma (mixed parotid tumour). This usually presents as a slowly growing, painless lump on the side of the face. If not completely excised it recurs and hence most surgeons advocate removing it with the whole of the surrounding superficial part of the gland (superficial parotidectomy). The facial nerve divides into a network in the substance of the gland and these tiny filaments have to be carefully traced and preserved.

Following parotidectomy a suction drain or Penrose drain with a pressure dressing is kept in position for several days to prevent haematoma formation. The facial nerve is checked to detect damage from surgery, and is checked subsequently for late damage (e.g. from a haematoma within the nerve sheath).

The lower face is likely to be swollen on the operated side making chewing and brushing the teeth difficult on that side. A soft diet and help with oral care is necessary until any oedema subsides.

Cancer

Cancer of the parotid is an uncommon and unpleasant disease as its extension to the base of the skull makes excision difficult or impossible.

Infections

In mumps the salivary glands are swollen and tender. Suppurative parotitis occurs in the severely debilitated if oral hygiene is inadequate.

Conditions of the Mouth

Injuries

Injuries to the mouth heal well, even if bone is exposed, because although the field is contaminated with saliva and mouth organisms, the blood supply is good and infection does not become established. However, healing is impaired and infection more likely after radiotherapy. Loss of tissue may well need plastic surgical procedures to minimize disfigurement and restore function. Lacerations of the tongue bleed profusely initially but heal readily; tongue movement during feeding results in sutures cutting out early and they are unnecessary even for extensive lacerations. When sutures are needed for reconstructive procedures, feeding via a nasogastric tube will reduce mouth movement.

Fractures of the lower jaw result in trismus and, if there is displacement, in non-alignment of the teeth. Treatment of these injuries is generally in the province of the dental surgeon who often will resort to immobilization of the jaws by interdental wiring. This holds the teeth of the upper and lower jaws together in the correct position while the fracture becomes stable.

NURSING CARE
The patient will need to have a special nurse for the first day and night. A nasopharyngeal tube is usually in position for up to 24 hours to facilitate the removal of secretions by suction. As the patient's jaws are fixed with wire there is little access to the airway. Wire cutters must be at hand; the surgeon will give precise instructions about when and where to cut the wires should airway obstruction occur. Anti-emetics are given to reduce the likelihood of vomiting. However, if the patient does vomit the nurse should first apply suction then, if necessary, cut the wires. The patient is nursed in the 'post-tonsillectomy position' (see Chapter 24, Fig. 24.4) until he is fully conscious when he can be gradually sat up.

Wiring the jaws together results in two other major nursing problems, which are the maintenance of a clean mouth and adequate nutrition.

Mouth care is needed at very frequent intervals initially. Once the patient is able to tolerate it the oral cavity may be irrigated using a weak sodium bicarbonate or chlorhexidine solution. As postoperative swelling subsides irrigation can be changed to mouth washes and a small toothbrush used on accessible areas of the teeth and gums. All visible wires must also be kept cleaned. The lips will quickly become dry and cracked unless a preparation such as Vaseline is frequently applied.

Most patients are able to commence an oral liquid diet by the second postoperative day. The services of a dietician may be required for a diet that is well balanced, sufficient in calories and palatable. If a liquidizer is available it should be used (this can allow the patient, with advice, to choose his own meals).

Writing materials must be available initially for communication. As the oedema subsides, articulation improves.

The wires remain in place for approximately 6 weeks. The patient must be competent at keeping his own mouth clean and be able to maintain adequate nutrition before discharge.

Halitosis

Halitosis is a common complaint and probably we all have bad breath from time to time. Common causes include particular dietary factors (e.g. curry or garlic), upper respiratory tract infection with purulent rhinorrhoea (particularly in children), and gingivitis. Gingivitis results in the collection of noisome material in pockets between the gums and the teeth. This may not be visible but massage of the gums with a cloth or toothpick yields the offensive smell. Gingivitis is due essentially to inadequate oral hygiene but dryness of the mouth from habitual mouth breathing is a contributory factor. Progression of gingivitis results in swelling of the gums and the loss of the interdental papillae followed by purulent discharge from the pockets around the teeth (pyorrhoea). Dental clearance (i.e. the extraction of all existing teeth) is most commonly carried out because of gingivitis. An unpleasant smell occurs where there is ulceration of the mouth or pharynx, particularly when due to carcinoma, or where there is extensive crusting of the nose, for example, in atrophic rhinitis.

Aphthous Ulceration

Aphthous ulceration of the mouth, of the Mickulicz type, is very common. These ulcers are elliptical or circular, a few millimetres in diameter, shallow and tender. They occur on the non-keratinizing epithelium of the mouth (see Chapter 21). They often occur in crops of two or three at a time and last about a week. Histologically, although the area of destruction is small, inflammation penetrates deeply, and if the under surface of the tongue is involved, movement of the tongue is so painful that there is dysphagia. These ulcers heal without scarring. There is a strongly inherited predisposition but the precise aetiology is unclear and they are not due simply to infection. The most effective treatment is probably to cover the tender area with a dental paste which will adhere to a moist surface: a topical steroid incorporated in the paste may aid healing (e.g. Adcortyl in Orabase). Other forms of aphthous ulceration are rare.

The Tongue

Repeated injury to the tongue or buccal mucosa from the teeth or dentures produces traumatic ulceration. So called furring of the tongue is of doubtful significance.

A black hairy tongue is due to infestation by pigmented micro-organisms between the papillae on the surface of the tongue and despite the alarming appearance, it is of no great importance. An effective remedy is to rub the tongue with fresh pineapple. The tongue may show areas of leukoplaka (white patches) which represent chronic epithelial change. Local areas of increased cell activity may be pre-cancerous but may be controlled by cryo-surgery or laser treatment. An ulcer of the tongue which fails to heal and which is not due to trauma, should be regarded as a carcinoma until proved otherwise.

24 Conditions of the Tonsils and Adenoids

TONSILLITIS IN CHILDREN

Incidence

The incidence of tonsillitis peaks at the age of 5 years, and again at the age of 10. This is reflected by enlargement of the tonsils to a maximum at the age of 5, followed by regression in size except for a slight increase at age 10.

Aetiology

Spread is by droplet infection, and cross-infection is particularly common between children starting school.

Pathology

The infecting organism may be a bacterium (usually the Streptococcus) or a virus (commonly the adenovirus, ECHO virus or influenza virus).

Symptoms

The child feels generally unwell, with a sore throat, difficulty swallowing, and sometimes referred earache (see Chapter 18). Very young children often do not complain of a sore throat, but will not eat.

Signs

Examination reveals a flushed, pyrexial child with enlarged, inflamed tonsils excluding pus and debris from their follicles

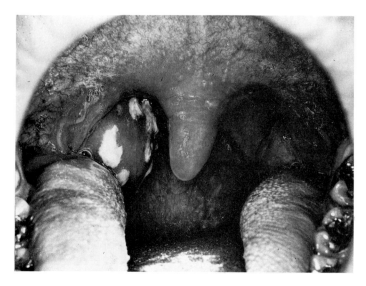

Fig. 24.1   Acute follicular tonsillitis.

(follicular tonsillitis) (Fig. 24.1). The cervical lymph nodes are enlarged and tender, especially the jugulodigastric node (tonsillar node) just below the angle of the mandible on each side.

Differential Diagnosis

Differential diagnosis is from infectious mononucleosis (glandular fever), agranulocytosis, Vincent's angina and, in the past, diphtheria. Scarlet fever is a streptococcal tonsillitis in which the bacteria produce a specific toxin which causes a punctate erythematous rash with circumoral pallor, and a 'strawberry and cream' tongue.

Investigations

Ideally a throat swab should be taken for culture and sensitivity.

The procedure must be explained to the patient. In order to counteract the natural inclination to lean back, the patient should be sat upright with his head against a firm surface. A child can sit upon his mother's (or a nurse's) lap with his feet tucked between her legs; a hand placed over the forehead keeps the head still,

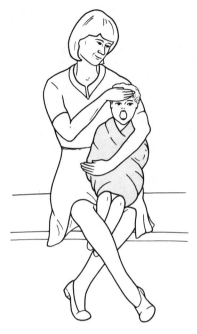

Fig. 24.2   Restraining a child for examination of the throat.

while the other hand secures the child's arms against his side, thus gently but effectively immobilizing him (Fig. 24.2).

A good light is essential so that the fauces can be clearly seen, and the swab is not contaminated from touching the mouth. In most patients it will be necessary to keep the tongue depressed with a spatula or depressor. Ask the patient to breathe through his mouth. The swab is quickly passed over the tonsils, picking up as much pus as possible; they should be swabbed firmly but the use of too much pressure should be avoided over the inflamed areas.

Treatment

Bed rest with plentiful oral fluids is advised; the sore throat is effectively relived by soluble paracetamol. Antibiotics should be withheld initially, on the basis that some infections are viral, and many bacterial infections naturally run a short, mild course. If, however, the child is no better after 24–48 hours, or if the throat swab grows a haemolytic streptococcus, then treatment with penicillin should be commenced. A satisfactory regime is penicillin V by mouth four times daily for 7 days. It is rarely necessary for a child suffering from tonsillitis to be admitted into hospital.

Complications

Complications include acute suppurative otitis media, quinsy, pharyngeal abscess, and the problem of recurrent tonsillitis.

TONSILLITIS IN ADULTS

Tonsillitis is less common after puberty, and it is necessary to beware of chronic pharyngitis as the real cause of a sore throat. Management is the same as for children.

QUINSY (PERITONSILLAR ABSCESS)

Aetiology

A quinsy develops when an episode of tonsillitis is complicated by spread of infection into the peritonsillar space, in close relationship to the upper pole of the tonsil; the result is a peritonsillar cellulitis which, if untreated, will progress to a peritonsillar abscess. The patient is usually a young adult.

Symptoms

Symptoms are initially those of acute tonsillitis, but after a few days the patient feels more ill and the sore throat becomes severe and unilateral, often with referred earache. Muscle spasm produces trismus (inability to fully open the mouth), and this coupled with the severity of the sore throat produces dysphagia, which may be so severe that the patient is unable to swallow even his own saliva.

Signs

The patient is clearly unwell and in pain, and is pyrexial. Trismus may make examination of the throat difficult, but even a limited

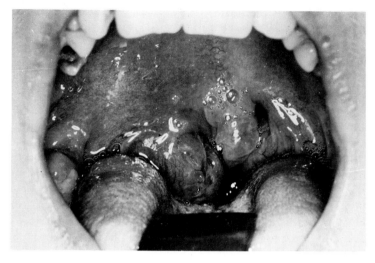

Fig. 24.3 A right quinsy.

view is sufficient to reveal gross swelling of the soft palate and anterior faucial pillar on the affected side, with displacement of the uvula across the midline towards the opposite side (Fig. 24.3).

Investigations

Investigations comprise a throat swab for culture and sensitivity, a full blood count and a Paul–Bunnell test to exclude infectious mononucleosis.

Treatment

In some patients there is clearly abscess formation with pus pointing, and the treatment is incision and drainage under topical anaesthesia with penicillin cover.

A record of all intake and output, and recordings of vital signs are commenced on admission, and continued for as long as is necessary.

Bed rest is maintained for several hours after incision. Regular thorough oral hygiene is essential throughout the stay in hospital.

Before incision and drainage is performed the patient will need to be given an explanation of the procedure. The most commonly used topical anaesthetic agents are cocaine 10% or lignocaine 4%.

This is applied by the doctor placing a small swab dipped in the solution against the area chosen for incision. The instrument used to incise a quinsy is a No 7 Bard–Parker handle with a No 15 guarded blade. The blade is guarded with a strip of adhesive tape 0.5 cm from the edge so that only the tip of the blade enters the tissues and adjacent structures are not damaged. Suction equipment with a Yankauer's pharyngeal sucker (disposable if possible) should be available.

Immediately prior to incision the patient should be helped into an upright position and be well supported with pillows. Night-wear must be protected; a receiver and tissues should be at hand.

A good light, tongue depressor, and spatula are essential aids during the incision. Immediately following incision the patient is helped to sit forward and encouraged to spit out the pus which will be draining into his mouth. A specimen will be taken for culture and sensitivity. When drainage of pus has ceased a mouth wash is given, the patient made as comfortable as possible and left to rest. A clean, covered receiver is left by the bedside. The relief from pain and trismus is rapid, but not immediate, and the patient may still need to spit out some saliva as well as pus for a while. A small amount of bleeding is to be expected following incision but this should rapidly subside.

Referred otalgia via the glossopharyngeal nerve is frequently present and analgesia will be required. There will still be some discomfort and dysphagia following incision but the relief from symptoms is such that oral fluids can be commenced within a few hours. The diet that can be offered, and tolerated, is gradually increased from fluid to solid.

Mobilization progresses as the patient's condition improves. As the majority of these patients are young, otherwise fit adults, recovery is usually rapid. The patient quickly becomes bored, especially when isolated and attempts to alleviate this must be made.

The patient is discharged once he is able to take adequate nourishment and has been apyrexial for 24 hours. This is usually before a course of antibiotics is complete.

On discharge the patient is given sufficient antibiotics to complete the course, and information about the need for tonsillectomy in the future. He should maintain regular, thorough oral hygiene, not attend work or school for at least 1 week, and keep any OPD appointment given.

In many cases however, abscess formation has not yet occurred when the patient presents in hospital, as the peritonsillar cellulitis has been partly suppressed by antibiotics prescribed by the GP. In this situation the patient is admitted and isolated in a single room; paracetamol is usually sufficient to control the pain, but sedation (e.g. with diazepam) may be needed. An intravenous infusion is set up, and benzyl penicillin is given intravenously every 6 hours; rapid resolution usually follows, and after 48 hours the patient may be changed to oral penicillin V to complete at least a 10 day course. The rate of improvement will regulate what can be drunk and eaten; as the cellulitis subsides pain will decrease and the diet can gradually be changed from fluid to solid. Frequent oral toilet is necessary. Mobilization starts as soon as the patient feels well enough. The combination of immobility and poor oral intake of fluids and solids may result in constipation; this is a problem which may be overlooked as it is uncommon in young adults on an ENT ward.

When the patient is ready to go home he will need to be given the same advice and information as a patient who has had a peritonsillar abscess incised.

When a patient has had a quinsy, tonsillectomy is advised as quinsies tend to recur. Most surgeons perform an interval tonsillectomy 6 weeks after resolution of the quinsy, but some prefer to operate at the time of the infection (quinsy tonsillectomy).

TONSILLECTOMY

Indications

In the past there has been much controversy over the indications for tonsillectomy. It is now appreciated, however, that the tonsils have a role in the immune defence of the body against infection, and that their removal is warranted only if they are causing more trouble than they are worth.

Recurrent tonsillitis is the most common indication for surgery; operation is advised if the patient has had three attacks a year or more in each of the last 2 years, or five attacks or more in the preceding year, with substantial loss of time from school or work. Other indications include a single quinsy, recurrent middle ear infection associated with tonsillitis, and unilateral tonsillar enlargement (which suggests the possibility of a neoplasm). The size of the tonsils is alone no reason for their removal, unless the swelling is unilateral as has just been mentioned, or unless they are so large as to cause respiratory obstruction in childhood.

Contra-indications

Contra-indications include tonsillitis or an upper respiratory tract infection within the 2 week period prior to operation, contact with one of the infectious diseases of childhood (especially measles), and a bleeding tendency or anaemia.

Operative Technique

The old technique of guillotine tonsillectomy has now largely been abandoned, and most surgeons remove the tonsils by dissection under general endotracheal anaesthesia, taking care to ensure haemostasis.

Nursing Management

Pre-operative Objectives

1 Ensure that there are no contra-indications to tonsillectomy.
2 Give the child and his parents adequate information about ward routine and pre-operative and postoperative events (e.g. expected length of stay).
3 Provide emotional and psychological support for the child and his parents.
4 Prepare the child for general anaesthesia.

Pre-operative Care

Hospitalization is a major event in anyone's life. This is especially so for children and their parents, and for many children tonsillectomy is their first planned admission to hospital. Preparation can start from the time the need for operation is explained to the child and his parents in the outpatient area. There are some excellent games available which can be employed in helping reduce the traumatic effects of hospitalization, and parents can be advised regarding their purchase. Space and family circumstances permitting, mothers should be encouraged to stay with their children, particularly those of pre-school age. Failing this, open visiting has proved to be of much value to the child, his family and the nursing staff.

The child is normally admitted to hospital the day before operation. Admission procedures vary but a specially devised questionnaire or nursing history sheet is usually employed. Essential questions include:

1 Those relevant to the contra-indications listed on p. 206.
2 Details of any loose teeth, which might be dislodged and inhaled in the operating theatre.
3 Specific likes and dislikes in food.
4 Special terms the child uses for toilet purposes.

Vital signs are taken and recorded. The child must be weighed as this is essential for drug dose calculation. A specimen of urine is collected for ward urinalysis and many older children find this particularly stressful. A specimen of blood is taken for haemoglobin estimation.

An explanation of the operation and the events surrounding it are given to the parents and child. The amount and depth of information given to the child must be appropriate for his age and stage of development. All questions asked by the child must be answered truthfully to gain his trust. The children on the ward are encouraged to play together before and after surgery.

The operation is performed under a general anaesthetic which requires the child to starve for several hours beforehand, necessitating a certain amount of vigilance from the nursing staff and mother. Drugs and routes used for premedication vary. Amongst the most commonly used are trimeprazine tartrate (Vallergan) and atropine sulphate, as both can be given by mouth.

In many wards small groups of children are nursed within a specific area after operation as this facilitates observation by the nursing staff and availability of emergency equipment. However, any changes in situation should be made before the child receives premedication and goes to theatre to reduce the psychological trauma of returning to unfamiliar surroundings.

The time the child spends in the operating department is the most stressful period for the parents and much support is required during this time. In particular it should be explained that there will be some delay after the operation before the child returns to the ward, because of time spent in the operating theatre recovery area.

208   *Chapter 24*

Postoperative Objectives

1 Maintain a clear airway.
2 Monitor vital signs and observe for signs of haemorrhage.
3 Maintain adequate hydration and nourishment.
4 Relieve discomfort and pain.
5 Promote healing of the tonsil beds.

Postoperative Care

Postoperative care must be of the highest quality; bleeding may be occult and rapidly fatal. On return to the ward the child can be nursed in either the traditional tonsillectomy position, which is three-quarters prone with the head turned to one side, or in the same position with one pillow under the chest (Fig. 24.4). Either method will aid the drainage of secretions and prevent the

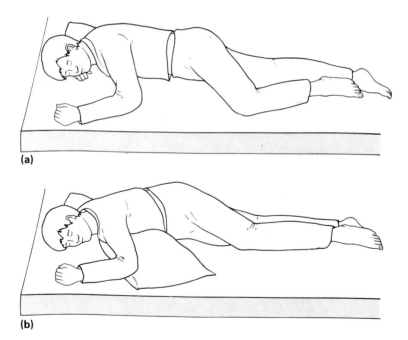

Fig. 24.4 Post-tonsillectomy position (the classical three-quarters prone, post-anaesthetic position); (b) modified post-tonsillectomy position: a pillow is placed under the child's chest to encourage any blood to drain down and out of the mouth rather than being swallowed.

aspiration of blood or vomit. Vital signs are recorded every 15 minutes initially, and then less frequently if they remain stable.

Haemorrhage is the most common complication; early signs are excessive swallowing and fresh blood, which may drain from the mouth or be vomited. Late signs are an increasing pulse rate, pallor and restlessness. Complaints of epigastric discomfort may indicate gastric irritation from swallowed blood. Procedures for the treatment of haemorrhage are given on p. 210. A slight elevation in the temperature is often present the day of operation and the day after, and is due to surgical trauma. A more marked elevation in temperature is due to lobar collapse or infection. The temperature should be recorded every 4 hours throughout the period of hospitalization.

When the child is sufficiently recovered from the anaesthetic, he can be given small amounts of iced water or fruit juice. This is gradually increased until he is able to tolerate a full diet. Most children are able to cope with a normal diet and a high fluid intake from the morning of the operation. Chewing and swallowing will help to increase salivary flow, reduce any spasm of the pharyngeal muscles and remove debris from the tonsil beds. After each meal and before going to bed the child should brush his teeth and rinse or gargle with a mouthwash, for example hydrogen peroxide, to keep the mouth and oropharynx as clean as possible.

Analgesics and sedatives are given as ordered. In the sedated child the nurse must be particularly thorough when observing for haemorrhage. A soluble analgesic, for example paracetamol, is given half an hour before meals to relieve the pain and discomfort of swallowing. Analgesics may also be required for referred otalgia (see Chapter 18). A distressed unhappy child gains much comfort from a cuddle.

In the absence of complications the child will be able to join in the general activities and play the day after surgery. Adequate rest is essential and a rest period in the afternoon is well accepted and used by all age groups.

When the child is ready to go home, usually 2–3 days after surgery, the parents need to be given some advice on care. The child should not return to school or crowded areas, for example cinemas, for 2 weeks. The afternoon rest period should continue for the first week at home; diet and oral hygiene should follow the same pattern as in hospital. An outpatient appointment may be given.

Tonsillectomy in Adults

The care that has been described for tonsillectomy, and the complications of tonsillectomy, in a child can be adapted for an adult as the nursing problems are similar. Adults frequently appear to suffer more pain and discomfort from referred otalgia than children.

Complications of Tonsillectomy

REACTIONARY HAEMORRHAGE
This may occur within the first 24 hours of operation, and is due to a vessel which went into spasm at the time of surgery subsequently relaxing and bleeding. Bleeding may be obvious, but sometimes the only indications are swallowing movements, 'rattly' breathing, and later a rising pulse. The throat must be examined under a good light, and all blood clot removed from the fossa which is bleeding; this alone may allow the tissues to retract and the bleeding to stop spontaneously. In the cooperative older patient, topical adrenaline may be applied to the tonsillar fossa on a swab. If bleeding persists, or is profuse, blood must be taken for haemoglobin, grouping and cross-matching, an intravenous infusion set up, and the patient returned to the operating theatre for ligation of the bleeding point.

On return to the ward the child is nursed in the same position as following tonsillectomy. Observations for haemorrhage and of vital signs are recorded every 15 minutes initially, then gradually reduced as the child's condition improves.

Fluid balance records are maintained until they are no longer necessary. Observations for incompatibility are made whilst any blood transfusion is in progress. The intravenous infusion is usually discontinued within 24 hours of the bleeding point being ligated. As the child is well hydrated during this time thirst is not a problem. When the child has sufficiently recovered, small amounts of oral fluids should be encouraged. Diet is gradually increased as his condition improves until solids can be tolerated.

Analgesics will be given and oral hygiene undertaken, as for tonsillectomy. The child will be able to get out of bed and join the ward activities when fit enough, which is usually by the second postoperative day.

Haemorrhage is a very frightening experience for the child and his parents, and the whole family will need much emotional and psychological support.

SECONDARY HAEMORRHAGE

This may occur between 5 and 10 days after the operation, and is due to infection of the tonsillar fossae. The bleeding takes place from granulation tissue and is seldom severe; removal of the clot, sedation in bed and treatment with a suitable antibiotic (e.g. amoxycillin), is usually all that is necessary.

Observations of vital signs are recorded. The interval between these observations varies according to the amount of bleeding. If the bleeding is slight (or, as is frequently the case, it stops following the removal of a clot) the child can be nursed sitting upright in bed rather than in the tonsillectomy position.

The child is given a covered receiver and tissues and asked to spit out any blood that may come from the tonsillar fossae rather than swallow it. If blood has been swallowed, epigastric pain and nausea may be present. Once the bleeding has stopped and the child is able, oral fluids and diet can be commenced. Regular and thorough oral hygiene, which includes brushing the teeth and gums, is essential.

As the child is likely to be discharged before the course of antibiotics is complete he will need to take the remainder home.

On rare occasions it is necessary to return the patient to the operating theatre to arrest the haemorrhage under general anaesthesia. In such cases the tonsillar fossae are extremely friable; ligation of bleeding points is impracticable, and the bleeding is controlled by suturing the faucial pillars together, possibly over a piece of Surgicel.

The care on return from theatre is similar to that following ligation of a bleeding point for reactionary haemorrhage. The patient is nursed in the same position and the same observations are carried out. Initially the throat is very sore. Dysphagia is likely, making it very difficult to swallow anything other than fluids for at least 24 hours.

ACUTE SUPPURATIVE OTITIS MEDIA

This sometimes occurs as a complication of tonsillectomy; intermittent referred earache is common after tonsillectomy, but persistent otalgia calls for an inspection of the tympanic membrane.

ADENOIDAL HYPERTROPHY

The adenoid lymphoid tissue enlarges to reach maximum size relative to the nasopharynx at about the age of three, and then steadily undergoes atrophy until by the late teens little or no adenoid tissue remains. In 3–6 year old children repeated upper respiratory tract infections can cause marked adenoidal hypertrophy, resulting in obstruction of the nasopharynx.

Clinical Features

Adenoidal hypertrophy results in nasal obstruction with mouth breathing and snoring, impaired speech and a high-arched palate, producing the appearance termed adenoid facies; rhinorrhoea and a post-nasal drip are common. Secondary sinusitis may develop, as may secretory otitis media, or recurrent acute suppurative otitis media. Examination confirms nasal obstruction, and posterior rhinoscopy demonstrates a large adenoid pad. If it is not possible to obtain a view of the post-nasal space, and adenoid hypertrophy is suspected, a soft-tissue lateral X-ray of the post-nasal space will outline the adenoid mass and demonstrate the size of the nasopharyngeal airway (Fig. 24.5).

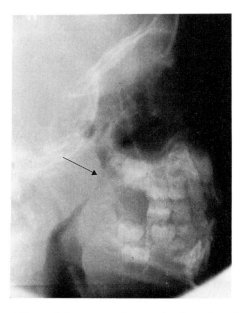

Fig. 24.5 Lateral X-ray of the post-nasal space, showing enlarged adenoids.

Treatment

If there is a marked degree of nasal obstruction, and particularly if there is associated otological disease, surgical removal of the adenoids is indicated. Children with cleft palate are an exception—the adenoids should not be removed because of the risk of causing a deterioration in speech. The indications for adenoidectomy are entirely separate from those for tonsillectomy, but nevertheless adenoidal hypertrophy commonly co-exists with recurrent tonsillitis, and so tonsillectomy and adenoidectomy are often carried out as a combined operation.

The operation of adenoidectomy is carried out under general endotracheal anaesthesia, the adenoid mass being removed with a curette. Postoperative care is similar to that for tonsillectomy, however, the throat will not be painful.

Complications

Reactionary haemorrhage, occuring within 24 hours of operation may require the insertion of a post-nasal pack under general anaesthesia; the pack is removed on the ward after 24 hours. Antibiotic cover is necessary to prevent local sepsis and acute otitis media.

The nursing care is similar to that described in Chapter 16 following insertion of a post-nasal pack for epistaxis. It will be necessary to explain to the child, and his parents, why the nose feels so blocked, and to ask the child not to touch the various tapes. There are many ways of keeping children content and occupied during the time that they are confined to bed. If their mothers are able to stay, they can be of great benefit to a child and the nursing staff by helping the child feel less insecure, miserable and unhappy.

Recurrence of adenoid tissue may follow incomplete removal.

OBSTRUCTIVE ENLARGEMENT OF THE TONSILS AND ADENOIDS

In some children, the tonsils and adenoids become so large that they interfere seriously with feeding and respiration (Fig. 24.5). Enlarged tonsils and adenoids can also be responsible for the *obstructive sleep apnoea syndrome*, in which there is loud snoring during sleep interrupted by frequent periods of obstructive apnoea. Chronic alveolar hypoventilation may progress to pulmonary hypertension and cor pulmonale, and there may be associated hypersomnolence, poor school performance, enuresis and delayed physical development. Treatment by adeno-tonsillectomy is immediately and dramatically effective.

25 Dysphagia and Dysphonia: Endoscopy

DYSPHAGIA

Difficulty in swallowing (dysphagia) is a serious symptom because it impairs the nutrition of the individual and also because all too commonly it is due to a sinister underlying cause.

Cleft Palate

If there is a palatal defect (e.g. as in congenital cleft palate) then on attempted swallowing, food and liquid is pushed into the nasal cavity from the mouth. A baby with this defect cannot suckle normally; he may need to be spoon fed with the aim of getting milk to the back of the mouth and into the oropharynx. With the aid of gravity this may well be successful, but early management is with a prosthetic plate to close off the fistula. With adjustments at frequent intervals, this plate can remould the bony architecture of the alveolus, aiding future surgical repair.

The child with a cleft lip and palate will need a variety of surgical procedures performed which may extend over several years. The care can be shared by a variety of disciplines including paediatricians, dental, plastic and ENT surgeons and speech therapists. The Health Visitor and/or Paediatric Community Nurse can give much psychological support and advice regarding physical care, particularly feeding, when the child is at home.

Feeding is obviously a problem particularly for parents who may be feeling guilty as well as anxious. Feeds need to be given slowly, and there are various devices which can be employed to aid feeding and prevent fluid going up into the nasal cavity. Some infants may manage with an ordinary teat with the hole slightly enlarged. As well as the prosthetic plate described, there are cleft palate teats available; these look like an ordinary teat with a rubber flange attached above the teat, to close off the defect in the palate. A cleft palate feeding spoon has a bump in the middle creating a gutter on either side. Breast feeding is difficult as it requires more suction and effort by the infant, and weight gain is the only indication that sufficient amounts are being taken. It can be successful when there is a cleft lip with normal palate.

The baby with a cleft lip and palate will swallow a lot of air during feeding necessitating frequent winding sessions.

About 60% of children with cleft palate have associated middle ear disease, with Eustachian tube dysfunction. Insertion of grommets is likely to be necessary. Regular examination of the ears, including audiometry, should not be neglected.

Fistulae into the nose or sinuses may also result from dental extraction or perforating injuries and may be closed by fashioning local flaps.

Foreign Bodies

Dysphagia also occurs if the pharynx is inflamed or paralysed or if a foreign body is impaled or impacted in the pharynx. In the majority of patients seen as an emergency with painful dysphagia after swallowing a foreign body, the symptom is due simply to bruising or scratching of the mucosa as the foreign body has passed through; these patients can generally manage to drink water with a little discomfort, whereas if the foreign body is still present, attempted swallowing usually causes much more obvious distress.

Carcinoma

The sensation of food sticking in the neck with progressive difficulty and loss of weight suggests a carcinoma of the laryngopharynx or upper oesophagus (see Chapter 27).

Dysphagia will occur if the tongue is immobile (from rigidity or paralysis) or if it is painful to move (e.g. from ulceration).

Pharyngeal Pouch

A pharyngeal pouch is an uncommon condition due to the pharyngeal mucosa herniating through the surrounding muscle fibres. Gradually the pouch increases in size. It generally presents in an elderly person who gives a story of regurgitation of food which has just been swallowed. The patient may say that he can empty the pouch by pressing on his neck. It seems to be caused by the cricopharyngeal sphincter contracting prematurely during swallowing. Treatment is by surgery if the symptoms warrant it.

Treatment: Surgical Excision

Pre-operative Care

The patient comes into hospital 1 or 2 days prior to surgery. Physical and psychological preparation will be necessary. As these patients are usually elderly there may be medical and nursing problems other than those due to the pharyngeal pouch. A history of recurrent chest infections due to aspiration of food and saliva is likely and may indicate the need for pre-operative and postoperative physiotherapy.

Explanation to the patient about the postoperative period should include information concerning the nasogastric tube, the wound dressing and drain, and the possibility of an intravenous infusion. As the pouch is excised via an incision in the neck (usually on the left side) it will be necessary for a male patient to shave on the morning of the operation.

Postoperative Care

On return from surgery, patients are nursed lying on their backs with one or two pillows under the head. Later, patients can be helped to sit up in bed, and if recovery is straightforward, can be helped out of bed the following day.

If either a corrugated or Penrose drain has been used a firm dressing will have been applied in theatre; if a suction drain has been employed instead then there will usually be no dressing. The dressing is usually removed by the second postoperative day when a lighter dressing can be applied. Sutures will be removed within 7 days. Drainage usually ceases within 3 days. The presence of saliva makes drainage secretions rather thick and sticky, like mucus; this would indicate fistula formation. Rarely air may leak from the hypopharynx through the repair into the soft tissues of the neck; this produces surgical emphysema, which has a characteristic 'bean bag' feel on palpation. In severe cases it can cause sufficient pressure on the respiratory tract to produce respiratory distress.

Vocal cord paralysis, which may be temporary or permanent, is another rare complication (see Chapters 24 and 25 for further information) and is caused by injuring the recurrent laryngeal nerve during the operation.

A nasogastric tube will be *in situ* and the patient will be fed by this route only for 4–5 days to allow the pharyngeal repair to heal. Unless the patient complains of nausea there is no need to aspirate the nasogastric tube until feeding commences. Most patients are able to tolerate nasogastric feeding within 24 hours of surgery and once feeding is established any intravenous infusion is removed.

A small amount of water coloured with methylene blue or Ribena is sometimes given before the nasogastric tube is removed. This is to test for fistula formation; if a fistula is present the coloured fluid will be seen to ooze through the drain site or from the suture line. If this does occur the nasogastric tube will remain until the fistula closes. In the absence of a fistula the tube is removed and fluids followed by a light soft diet, can be given. Very firm solid food, for example grilled chops, should be avoided for a while until the pharyngeal repair has strengthened. The patient is usually delighted with the relief from regurgitation and dysphagia.

Particular care will need to be paid to oral hygiene for as long as the nasogastric tube is *in situ*.

Diathermy Coagulation

If the patient is unfit for excision of the pouch then division of the septum between the pouch and oesophagus by diathermy (Dohlman's operation) can be performed via a special oesophagoscope. The psychological and physical preparation is similar. A nasogastric tube will be in position for 4–5 days following the treatment before oral feeding is attempted. Fistula formation is not a problem following this procedure but surgical emphysema and mediastinal abscess have been known to occur.

Achalasia

At the lower end of the oesophagus failure of the cardiac sphincter to relax on swallowing (achalasia of the cardia) produces dysphagia occurring in a younger age group—good results may follow surgical division of the sphincter (Heller's operation).

Oesophageal Stricture

Benign oesophageal stricture may follow reflux oesophagitis from incompetence of the cardiac sphincter, whereby acid stomach contents are regurgitated into the oesophagus. Such strictures may also result from swallowing corrosive fluids; they may be managed by repeated dilation (which carries the risk of oesophageal rupture), or by resection and reconstruction.

Complications

Wherever there is dysphagia, particularly where there is dysfunction of the pharynx, there is concern that saliva and other material may be inhaled from the pool in the pharynx (spillover). This may present in the early stage as cough on lying down. Later complications are pulmonary collapse and lung abscess.

DYSPHONIA

The vocal sound is produced by the vocal cords. These are set into vibration by air passing between them when they are adducted (brought together). The regulation of tightness of the cords and the breath pressure is balanced in such a way that the column of air is interrupted, the interruptions occurring at high frequency (for example, as in an oboe, or as the noise children make when blowing between blades of grass). The tightness (and possibly the bulk) of the cords and the pressure of the expired air control the *pitch* and the *loudness* of the voice.

The quality of the voice depends on the shape and size of the resonating cavities in the head, chiefly the oropharynx. Consonants are added by movements of the lips, tongue and soft palate.

Disorders of the Voice

Excessive use of the voice, for example the shouting of football supporters, produces hoarseness and discomfort when talking. The excessive friction results in an excess of mucus production which itself induces repeated clearing of the throat with a shallow cough (frog in the throat). This itself produces slight trauma and tends to perpetuate the condition. In the more florid case there are small areas of haemorrhage and oedema and if this is not allowed to recover by vocal rest, permanent structural changes occur which account for the characteristic vocal qualities of some pop singers. The slightest irregularity of the edge of the vocal cords alters the voice quality and benign or malignant change here presents early. Hoarseness due to oedema of the cords is a feature of thyroid dysfunction, and a painful hoarse voice is a feature of acute laryngitis, generally following an upper respiratory tract infection.

Muscle dysfunction producing dysphonia occurs in Parkinsonism, myasthenia gravis and in recurrent laryngeal nerve palsy.

Inability to close off the nasal cavity posteriorly (e.g. from cleft palate) results in the escape of air via the nose on talking. 'Explosive' consonants (in which pressure is built up in the mouth of pharynx and then released suddenly, as in making the sound 'K' or 'P') are particularly affected. Conversely, obstruction of the nasal airway, for example by adenoids or nasal polypi, affects the voice in a characteristic way (which the reader can mimic by speaking while holding the nose closed).

In many patients referred because of dysphonia, the structures are normal and the problem is a psychogenic one. Commonly the patient has no voice and it is found on examination that the cords look normal but do not come together on attempted phonation. However, the patient can cough normally.

ENDOSCOPY

Endoscopy is the examination of hollow viscera or body cavities using an inspecting instrument passed either through a stab incision or via one of the natural orifices. Endoscopes may be straight and rigid, or flexible. A rigid endoscope is needed if a foreign body has to be removed or if a sizeable biopsy is to be taken; the surgeon looks along the instrument and can grasp the foreign body under direct vision using special forceps passed along the endoscope. As these hard rigid endoscopes are passed through the mouth it is important that any dental prosthesis is removed and the presence of any loose or crowned tooth noted. If inspection only is required, a rigid endoscope with magnification (the Hopkin's rod) gives a splendid view where it can be used (e.g. of the larynx or pharynx when passed via the mouth, or of the trachea and inferior aspect of the larynx via a tracheostomy if present, or of the TM via the external canal).

A flexible endoscope is made of a bundle of tiny glass fibres. These fibres are so fine that they can be made to bend and curve without breaking. Light can travel down the bundle because the rays of light (which of course travel in straight lines) are reflected repeatedly from the walls of the individual fibres. Such an endoscope carries several hundred fibres, each one transmitting a view of a small area of the visual field and so a composite picture is produced. The flexible instrument can be inserted via a nostril, preferably after topical anaesthetic has been sprayed into the nasal fossa. (It may be also more comfortable if the patient is given a decicaine or amethocaine lozenge to suck or 5 ml of xylocaine gel to hold in the mouth and swallow.) The coiled cable has a plug at its free end for connection to a special fibroptic light source. The hand piece is equipped with a finger-operated control which bends the tip of the endoscope—shown bent upwards in the photograph—this determines the view obtained and directs the endoscope as it is passed. To avoid 'fogging' by the patients warm breath condensing on the instrument and obstructing the view, the tip may be initially dipped in 'Savlon' (chlorhexidine). As the instrument passes through the nose the nasal cavity can be inspected. Because this part of the respiratory tract is rigid, a good view is seen. As the instrument is gently advanced, it comes to lie on the soft palate. The tip needs to be bent to see into the pharynx. With the patient breathing through the nose, the laryngeal inlet and the vocal cords can be seen. But with the endoscope in this position, movements of the soft palate on swallowing and on phonation can be inspected—of value in assessing the results of cleft palate repair, for example. Keeping the larynx in view, the endoscope can be advanced further down the pharynx to obtain close-up views of the structures. In more complicated endoscopes, there are also channels for suction, washing and for instruments carrying tiny biopsy forceps on the end of wires. Such flexible endoscopes have three important advantages:

1 they can be used without the patient needing a general anaesthetic and are thus suitable for outpatient procedures, economizing in hospital accommodation;

2 because they can negotiate corners, they can therefore inspect recesses which would otherwise be obscured, for example suitable

instruments can inspect the stomach and small and large bowel and the divisions of the bronchial tree. Similarly they are of great value where normally a rigid endoscope would be used but this is rendered impossible by virtue of trismus or neck rigidity.

3   If the patient is conscious, the movements of structures under voluntary control (e.g. soft palate, larynx and pharynx) can be examined and, if a camera is attached, recorded.

Endoscopic Procedures

In ENT surgery, the endoscopic procedures to be considered are:
    Antroscopy
    Nasendoscopy
    Pharyngoscopy
    Laryngoscopy
    Bronchoscopy
    Oesophagoscopy.

Antroscopy

Antroscopy is the inspection of the maxillary antrum, via a hole made in the medial wall of the antrum (as in performing an antral lavage except that a larger trocar is used which can accommodate the endoscope).

Nasendoscopy

Nasendoscopy is now generally carried out using a flexible fibroptic endoscope (Fig. 25.1). Through this slender cable it is possible to inspect in detail the cavities of the nasal fossae. The movements of the soft palate and nasopharyngeal sphincter can be seen and recorded; this is of particular value where the functions of these parts have been affected by disease or by previous surgery.

Pharyngoscopy and Laryngoscopy

If the fibroptic nasendoscope is advanced into the nasopharynx and the tip directed downwards, the pharynx and larynx can be inspected. They may also be inspected under general anaesthesia using a rigid tube passed through the mouth (Fig. 25.1). Following this procedure the patient is nursed in the position he finds most

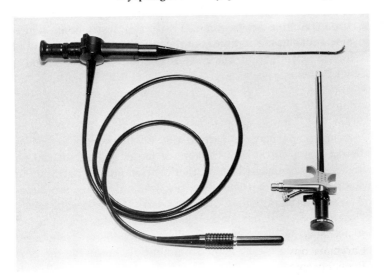

Fig. 25.1 This figure shows two instruments in increasingly common use. A pharyngoscope (the flexible instrument), and a rigid endoscope incorporating a Hopkin's rod lens.

comfortable. The examination and the taking of biopsies may cause oedema leading to stridor and obstruction—hence it is important to observe the rate, depth and sound of respirations in the early postoperative period. An emergency tracheostomy set, suction and oxygen must be available.

The pharynx may have been sprayed with a local anaesthetic. This will temporarily abolish the swallowing reflex so the patient is given nothing by mouth until 4 hours after the procedure to allow the effects of the local anaesthetic to wear off.

When a biopsy has been taken, especially from the vocal cords, use of the voice, including whispering, may be forbidden for 48 hours. The patient and his family should be advised about the need for this before the examination, and writing materials should be provided.

Bronchoscopy

The major bronchi can be inspected using rigid bronchoscopes and a variety of sizes is available for children and babies. Because of its flexibility, the use of a fibroptic instrument enables much more of the bronchial tree to be seen. Using this instrument, limited biopsies, brushings or scrapings of the mucosa may be obtained for cytological examination but it is unsuitable for the removal of foreign bodies.

Oesophagoscopy

Oesophagoscopy may be carried out on the conscious sedated patient using a fibroptic instrument or under general anaesthesia using a rigid oesophagoscope. Either instrument may perforate the oesophagus; this is particularly a risk when strictures are dilated and when foreign bodies are removed. If the oesophagus is perforated where it lies in the chest, there is the risk of a fatal mediastinitis. If the condition allows, immediate oesophageal repair via a thoracotomy is the treatment of choice. On the other hand, a perforation of the cervical oesophagus can often be managed conservatively.

The nurse must be aware of the possibility of perforation and must look for the signs and symptoms of it. These include pyrexia, tachycardia, hypotension, dyspnoea, pain (at the site of the perforation or referred to the shoulder blades) and surgical emphysema in the neck. The patient may look shocked and the skin is cold and clammy. Should a perforation be suspected, it must immediately be reported to the doctor.

Following oesophagoscopy the patient is not given anything by mouth for at least 6 hours, fluids are then permitted for 12 hours then a soft diet is introduced. Some surgeons prefer that a chest X-ray is taken before the diet is recommenced.

The oesophagoscope is marked in centimetres along its length and when in position, the distance of the tip of the oesophagoscope from the upper teeth or gums can be measured. Note that the site of a biopsy may thus be recorded as 30 cm for example, although the average length of the adult oesophagus is only 25 cm.

26 Stridor, Tracheostomy, Recurrent Laryngeal Palsy

STRIDOR

Stridor is an intermittent harsh sound in time with respiration and indicates airway obstruction. When heard only on inspiration the site of the obstruction is supraglottic (i.e. above the vocal cords); if on expiration (when the bronchus normally becomes narrower) it is intrathoracic, while if heard in both phases of respiration it may well be in the trachea.

Croup is an alarming barking cough and is due to narrowing of the larynx.

Laryngotracheobronchitis

Croup, together with stridor and hoarseness, is a feature of laryngotracheobronchitis when it occurs in a 6 month to 3 year old infant. This is a disease of viral origin following an upper respiratory tract infection (URTI). There is substernal recession and the child (and parents) are anxious and distressed. It is probably wise to admit such a child under 1 year of age. He may be given humidified oxygen and, uncommonly, tracheostomy or tracheal intubation may be required.

Epiglottitis

Epiglottitis generally presents in late infancy and childhood. It is an uncommon but dangerous condition with life threatened within hours of the onset of symptoms. There is a severe sore throat with dysphagia and then dribbling saliva. The epiglottis becomes swollen with oedema and obstructs the laryngeal inlet. An expert anaesthetist may be able to pass an endotracheal tube but a surgeon must be standing by to carry out immediate tracheostomy if the attempt fails. In many cases emergency tracheostomy is the treatment of choice, though once the child is on appropriate antibiotic treatment, generally chloramphenicol (the infection being treated by Haemophilis), there is rapid recovery within 1–2 days.

Trauma

Injury of the airway producing oedema and stridor is a feared consequence of inhalation of smoke or steam. (Children may inhale steam from the spout of a boiling kettle.)

Congenital Laryngeal Stridor

The commonest cause of chronic stridor is so called congenital laryngeal stridor. This appears soon after birth and generally recovers spontaneously in 2 years or so. The baby has marked inspiratory stridor brought on particularly with crying or excitement; the stridor disappears on sleep. The mechanism here is that the laryngeal inlet tends to close on inspiration and possibly neuromuscular coordination is at fault—when examined under anaesthesia the airway is seen to improve as the plane of the anaesthesia deepens. These children appear well and although the symptom is alarming, reassurance can be safely given.

Stridor is also a feature in the baby with a small lower jaw (Pierre Robin syndrome) where the tongue is held posteriorly and impedes the airway. Here again the problem generally resolves spontaneously but advice about nursing care may be given. Other defects, for example cleft palate, co-exist.

Other causes include subglottic stenosis, compression of the trachea from vascular anomaly (the right subclavian artery passing behind the trachea), stenosis of larynx or trachea from trauma (either direct injury or as a consequence of using endotracheal or tracheostomy tubes).

TRACHEOSTOMY

Tracheostomy is the making of a hole in the trachea. Generally this is kept open in the early postoperative phase by a tracheostomy tube, of which there are several types.

It is preferable to carry out the operation under general anaesthesia with an endotracheal tube in place. This method is impracticable if obstruction prevents the passing of the tube through the larynx into the trachea, in which case local anaesthesia may be needed. After making a skin incision (usually transverse) the underlying muscles are separated to reveal the anterior surface of the trachea. When the exposure is adequate, a hole is cut in the trachea, generally through the second and third tracheal rings. Suction is used to prevent aspiration of blood at this stage and the anaesthetist's tube, if present, is withdrawn. The tracheostomy tube is inserted and held in position either by suturing the flanges to the skin or by tying tapes around the neck.

The edges of the incision are lightly apposed. If the tracheostomy tube comes out inadvertently within 2 days or so of the operation, before a track has formed, the situation may quickly become desperate—the trachea is difficult to re-cannulate because the patient is 'fighting for breath' and with these movements the trachea moves up and down in the depths of a bloody hole making the stoma in the trachea difficult, if not impossible, to find. In order to avoid this, one practice has been to suture the anterior tracheal wall (or a flap of it) to the skin or subcutaneous tissues. However this may lead to subsequent tracheal stenosis. A better technique is to leave firm sutures through the trachea at the stoma site; these 'stay' sutures are left long, brought out through the wound and can be used to steady the trachea if early urgent re-cannulation becomes necessary.

Tracheostomy may be carried out for the reasons given below.
1 To protect the lungs from overspill (p. 245).
2 To bypass obstruction of the upper airway. Such obstruction may be, for example, due to inflammation with oedema, or to injury to neck or face. Similarly it may be done as a preliminary to operations on the face which themselves would result in respiratory obstruction.
3 To allow for positive pressure respiration, for example where there is inadequate chest movement (from injury or paralysis).
4 As part of a laryngectomy operation, where a permanent tracheostomy is fashioned.
In some of these situations it may be possible to use an indwelling endotracheal tube as an alternative, but this runs the increased risk of producing ulceration of the mucosa and necrosis of the tracheal cartilage with subsequent stenosis. If the airway needs to be

artificially maintained for longer than a few days, probably a tracheostomy is to be preferred. (In children the Jackson–Rees endotracheal tube has been used for periods of a few weeks without untoward sequelae.) Tracheostomy has its own risks of causing subsequent stenosis either from collapse at the site of the stoma or at a lower level from necrosis and resulting fibrosis at the site of the cuff. In recent years the increasing use of the low pressure, high volume ('floppy') cuff has reduced this latter problem.

Tracheostomy is often an emergency operation and may need to be performed under local anaesthetic or with no anaesthesia to be life saving. In an emergency a large bore needle or cannula may be pushed through the skin into the trachea.

Pre-operative Nursing Care

Whenever possible the operation is performed under a general anaesthetic, and the patient is prepared for this as described in Chapter 1. The neck skin is prepared as necessary. It is essential that the patient and his family are given as full an explanation of the operation as is possible in individual circumstances. This should include information about the site of the opening, the tube, tracheal suction, humidification and when possible the planned duration of the tracheostomy. Generally it is helpful if the patient can see and handle the equipment to be used. If the patient is to be nursed postoperatively in an intensive therapy unit it may reduce anxiety if he visits the area prior to the operation.

The anticipated loss of speech is very frightening and one of the most worrying aspects is the fear of being alone and unable to call for attention. Even fully conscious adult patients will need one nurse to care for them in the initial postoperative period and should be reassured that they will not be left alone. Pen, paper and call-bell can be seen to be available before the operation. If there is time, various non-verbal communication signs can be practised. If the patient is illiterate, picture card signs are useful, and these can quite easily be made by sticking pictures from nursing and other magazines onto pieces of cardboard.

Many members of the health care team are involved in the care of these patients. The nurse has more contact with the patient, and his family, than others and will need to be able to reinforce and, on occasion, clarify explanation given by others.

The pre-operative care for laryngectomy is described in Chapter 27.

Postoperative Care

Before the patient returns to the area the following equipment needs to be checked and made available:

Suction equipment, catheters and gloves.

Humidification equipment.

Tracheal dilators.

Spare tracheostomy tube with introducer and tapes.

Lubrication for the spare tube, if used.

Oxygen.

Call bell.

Communication materials.

If the tape and size of tube are not known until the patient returns from theatre the spare tube must be made available as quickly as possible. Other items may be necessary depending on the reason for the tracheostomy, for example a mechanical ventilator. The nursing problems which are present following tracheostomy arise from the upper respiratory tract being bypassed and the resulting inability to cough and speak, and to warm, moisten and filter incoming gases. Much of the care of these patients is based on attempting to replace or compensate the effects of losing these functions.

Loss of Speech

It can be both frightening and frustrating to be unable to communicate verbally. When communication is limited to writing only, it becomes a time consuming and tiring task. Some patients may not be able to write. These are difficult concepts for anyone to fully appreciate, even if the voice has been lost from laryngitis for a short time.

It is important to remember that the patient's previous hearing levels have not altered. There is no need for anyone to either shout or write down information. If a hearing aid was worn before tracheostomy it should be in good working order and worn after the operation. If the patient can write, allow him sufficient time to do so, and take time to actually read what has been written, and when necessary and appropriate, 'read between the lines'.

It is difficult to communicate depth of feelings such as fear or worry by the written word alone, unless one is gifted or practised. Some indication can be gained by observing facial expression, hand and body movements and the other forms of non-verbal communication that are employed to supplement and reinforce oral communication. Magic slates are useful as it is easy to remove what has been written on them; one does not like to be reminded of what one has said in certain circumstances and the same applies when writing is the only available means of communication! No-one should ever intrude upon a patient's privacy by reading, without invitation, anything that has been written during a previous communication. Nurses caring for patients following tracheostomies can become quite skilled at lip reading, which eases the burden on the patient considerably.

It can take much patience, understanding and tact from the nursing staff to establish and maintain two-way effective communication but every effort must be made as it is essential for the patient's mental and physical well-being.

Loss of Upper Respiratory Tract Humidification

When gases are inspired through the nose they reach the trachea at approximately 32°C with a relative humidity of 98%. Breathing cold, dry air straight into the trachea results in drying of tracheal secretions and paralysis of the cilia which help in the removal of secretions and debris. Thus thick, dry secretions can accumulate to form crusts which predispose to infection and may block the tracheostomy tube. It is therefore essential to have some form of humidification and this is particularly important during the first few postoperative days. The most efficient humidifiers are those which allow all inspired gas to pass over heated water; however this equipment restricts the mobility of the patient so these humidifiers may only be used during the immediate postoperative period (24–48 hours) and subsequently during the night. There are various small disposable humidifiers which can be attached to the tube; they are quite effective but can be cumbersome for the fully mobile patient to wear. A simple but effective method of giving humidification is to tie a moist gauze swab around the neck in front of the tube with tape or ribbon gauze (Fig. 26.1). It is important that the gauze is kept moist but not dripping wet. This can be done by frequently spraying the area of gauze in front of the

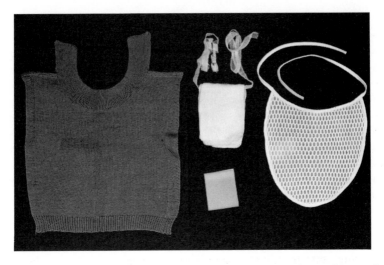

Fig. 26.1   Protectors/humidifiers. The Romet, gauze square, laryngofoam and Buchanan bibs.

tube opening with normal saline from a Rogers' crystal spray. The gauze must be changed frequently or it will act as a focus for infection. Spraying and changing the gauze can be done by many patients for themselves once they have been shown how to do this and appreciate its importance.

Also illustrated in Fig. 26.1 are the Romet and Buchanan bibs and the laryngofoam protector. The Romet bib is made of cotton, looks like a crew-neck sweater insert, and is available in eight colours. The white Buchanan bib is made of two layers of string vest cotton knit with a thin layer of foam in between. It is available on prescription and can be washed up to nine times. The laryngofoam protector is a small piece of foam with a strip of adhesive attached to one end. It is disposable, and available on prescription. It is quite small and therefore inconspicuous, and is possibly best suited to the laryngectomy patient who does not wear a tube or who has a stomal button.

Many patients like to wear these bibs over a gauze swab or laryngofoam protector as these protect the bib from direct contact with secretions. These bibs have much to offer from a cosmetic point of view as well as acting as filters and humidifiers.

Loss of Cough

Excessive secretions are moved up into the trachea by ciliary action and expelled by coughing. In order to cough, a deep breath is taken in and then forcibly compressed against closed vocal cords. When the cords open, the air which has been compressed inside the chest is forced upwards through the cords taking secretions and debris with it into the pharynx and sometimes the mouth. Following tracheostomy it is not possible to built up pressure in the chest because the air escapes through the tracheostomy tube. Secretions and debris will need to be removed by tracheal suction. The frequency and depth of suction required will vary with each patient. The patient can help by making limited coughing actions which will bring the secretions up to the tracheostomy tube, so that deep suction is rarely necessary. In time the patient can be taught to cough the secretions up into the pharynx or through the tube by temporarily occluding the end of the tube after breathing in. Occluding the tube permits an increase in intrathoracic pressure which can be used to produce a cough when the occlusion is removed. A clean finger covered by a disposable glove or piece of gauze can be used to occlude the tube.

   Obviously it is easier for thin secretions to move, and be removed, than thick tenacious secretions. Physiotherapy also plays an important part in keeping the lungs clear.

TRACHEAL SUCTION

Tracheal suction is an unpleasant procedure. Always give the patient an explanation of what you are about to do even if he has experienced suction before. Patients have been known to comment on the fact that the amount of distress and discomfort they experience is related to the individual who performs the procedure. It is important to be as gentle as possible to avoid damaging delicate tracheal lining and causing pain. Performing the procedure can be very frightening for a nurse, who should not be expected to do so before sufficient clinical demonstrations have been given. The principles of tracheal suction are as follows:

1   A clean technique is essential to avoid introducing infection. The portion of the catheter which is inserted into the trachea must remain sterile until insertion. There is no need to lubricate the tip of the catheter. A fresh catheter must be used for each insertion into the trachea.

2 If the patient is able to cough secretions as far as the end of the tracheostomy tube then the catheter need only be inserted just beyond the end of the tube. If in doubt about the length of the tube, look at the spare tube which is available for that patient. If the left bronchus requires suctioning special angle-tipped catheters are available for this purpose; a straight catheter invariably enters the right main bronchus as it is wider and more vertical than the left.

3 The catheter should be no wider than half the diameter of the tracheostomy tube to allow room for air to pass around it. If the catheter is too wide it will draw air out of the lungs more quickly than it is replaced, resulting in collapse of all or part of the lung (atelectasis).

4 The vacuum reading on the suction apparatus should be kept at low to medium on the gauge (up to 100 mm Hg for a child and 200 mm Hg for an adult). Too high a pressure can cause the catheter to collapse or adhere to the tracheal wall causing considerable damage to the mucosal lining. Suction must never be applied when the catheter is being introduced into the trachea, but only on withdrawal. The mucosa can be protected from suction catheter damage by using air-flo catheters. These have a special tip which prevents the holes of the catheter coming in contact with the tracheal mucosa.

5 Insertion, application of suction, and removal of catheter should be done within 10–15 seconds. Timing the procedure by holding your own breath as long as possible is not a very good guide as most nurses have a normal and healthy respiratory tract, unlike the patient. Allow the patient to rest between each application of suction.

6 The quantity and type of secretions being aspirated should be recorded. Specimens for culture and sensitivity can be taken as necessary using a sputum trap in-line to the suction apparatus (Fig. 26.2).

Wound Infection

The skin wound made at the time of tracheostomy requires care using an aseptic technique. Not only can it become infected like a wound in any other part of the body, but secretions from the trachea can collect around the outside of the tube and crusts can form. The wound is protected from the tube flanges by a dressing.

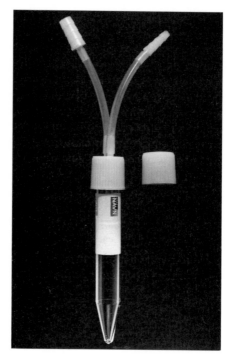

Fig. 26.2   A sputum trap.

Figure 26.3 shows two of the many prepacked sterile dressings available for this purpose. The dressing is changed at least once daily. After the dirty dressing is removed the stoma and wound area are cleaned before a clean dressing is applied. Dental rolls held in artery forceps are useful; as the roll protrudes past the hard tip of the forceps there is no possibility of the forceps ends coming in contact with the wound area. Cotton wool dressed applicators are useful for children and adolescents when forceps may be too large to fit comfortably and safely under the tube flanges. Whichever material is used must be well wrung out to prevent fluid trickling down into the trachea and causing a bout of coughing. Tilley's forceps are very useful for removing crusts from around the stoma. Sutures are removed according to instructions, usually about 5 days after surgery.

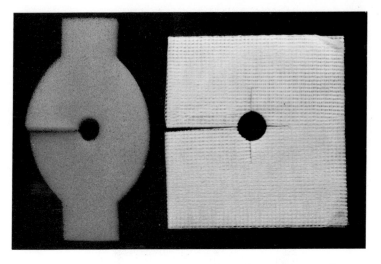

Fig. 26.3 The Shah foam tracheostomy dressing and a gauze type tracheostomy dressing.

Changing the Tracheostomy Tube

Following tracheostomy it takes 5–7 days for a track to form, and until this time has passed there is the danger of the tube being displaced or reinserted into the pretracheal tissues. The first tube change is often done by medical and nursing staff approximately 48 hours after surgery. The frequency of subsequent changes (which are done by nurses) varies with the nature of the secretions and the type of tube *in situ*. Two people are required to change a tracheostomy tube: one person removes the dirty tube using a curved, downward movement and the other immediately inserts the clean tube. Tracheal dilators must always be available.

Tapes are changed daily and two people are needed: one person to change the tapes, the other to hold the tube in place lest it should be coughed out. Tapes should be tied in a reef knot at each side of the neck (Fig. 26.4); it is more awkward to tie the knots at the back and this is in any case more uncomfortable for the patient. Tapes should be tied with the head flexed as it is in this position that the circumference of the neck is least. The tapes should just allow one finger to slide under them to ensure that they are firm but not too tight. If the tapes are of a different colour from white dressing materials, for example blue or green, they will be much

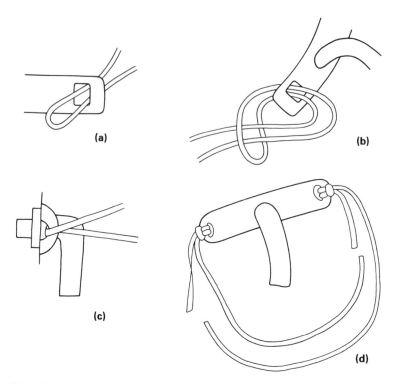

Fig. 26.4 A method of tying tapes on a tracheostomy or laryngectomy tube. (a) Loop tape through eyelet of flange, allowing one tape end to be longer than the other; (b) insert loose tape ends through loop; (c) draw the loose ends of the tapes firmly in place; (d) when the tube is in place tie a reef knot on each side of the neck, so as they are visible, using the ends of the short and long tapes. Cut off excess of tape. Finally check for security.

less likely to be accidentally cut. Tapes should not be tied in a bow as this can quite easily become undone and it can also be mistaken for a tie on the patient's nightwear.

If the patient is to go home with a tube *in situ* he must be taught all aspects of its care. A suction pump must be supplied for the patient to use at home. Relatives must also be aware of what is involved and why it is necessary. Additional care and support should be provided by the Community Nurse.

Removal of the Tube (Decannualtion)

On some occasions in adults the tube can be removed without any preliminaries. At other times (and always in children) the patient is gradually introduced to using the upper respiratory tract again. This can be done by:

1 Using a fenestrated tube (p. 245) in conjunction with a speaking valve. This fenestration allows the patient to breathe in through the tube and out through the larynx, and enables him to speak. Eventually the tube may be occluded by a special blocker and finally removed. This method is particularly applicable to children.

2 Inserting a smaller tube at each tube change. A smaller tube will allow more air to pass around it and the tracheostomy opening to gradually decrease in size.

3 Occluding the proximal end of the tube by a 'cork' so that ultimately the patient is not breathing through the tube at all and can sleep with the tube fully corked.

The patient will require close observation for respiratory distress irrespective of the method used.

Following removal of the tube an airtight dressing should be firmly applied to ensure that the patient is not breathing through the tracheostomy opening. If the patient is breathing through the opening and dressing, it may be some time before it becomes obvious that he still requires a tracheostomy for adequate ventilation. If the dressing is airtight, respiratory distress will occur earlier when there is still a reasonably sized opening for tube insertion. The stoma normally shrinks rapidly following decannulation and closes off spontaneously. The spare tube, tracheal dilators and suction equipment must be kept at hand until it is certain that they will no longer be needed.

Psychological Care

Psychological care starts as soon as the patient becomes aware of the need for tracheostomy and its effects. It is felt by some that loss of speech and tracheal suction have to be experienced to be truly appreciated. However, every effort must be made to ensure that the patient and his family are well prepared and informed, and as free from anxiety as possible.

Being unable to speak even for a short length of time can make the patient depressed, withdrawn or demanding. In Stockwell (1981) some of the nurses interviewed give poor communication and demanding behaviour as some of the reasons for their not enjoying looking after certain patients. If the patient is acting in any of these ways efforts should be made to find out why, and how he can be helped.

Nurses sometimes express their own fears about caring for a patient with a tracheostomy. These fears are mostly related to the unpleasantness of suction, the possibility of tube displacement, and the inability of the patient to communicate adequately. The nurse will also need to be allowed to express her concerns and be given enough knowledge, supervised practise and support for her to gain confidence and enjoyment when caring for these patients.

The patient will have to make many adjustments, particularly to his self perception, as his body has been altered. Some people may find their tracheostomy quite repulsive and difficult to accept. If a nurse shows revulsion towards the tracheostomy this will reinforce the patient's own feelings. By involving the patient in his own care one can help him to accept his altered self.

Some people feel that while they have a tracheostomy they are 'sick' and will act in a way that they feel is appropriate for a sick person to act, for example by being helpless or unable to make a decision. Family and friends may have similar attitudes. A visit from someone who is coping well with a tracheostomy may be of some help.

There may be changes in a patient's sleep pattern, for example the need for suction can prevent him getting adequate rest and may result in behaviour change. It is seldom necessary for a patient to be continuously nursed in the upright position following tracheostomy; during the night he may lie flat.

The patient and his family must together be involved if psychological needs are to be met following tracheostomy.

Nursing Management of Complications Following Tracheostomy

Haemorrhage

Haemorrhage can be primary, reactionary or secondary. If it is occurring from the wound site, pressure should be applied to control the bleeding. This is not always easy as the tube flanges may obstruct access to the bleeding point. Massive fatal haemorrhage can occur from erosion of a major vessel by the tube. If not already in position a cuffed tube should be inserted; by inflating the cuff, pressure will be applied which can help control bleeding from within or around the trachea, as well as prevent aspiration of blood coming from any point above the cuff.

Blockage of the Tube

Regular changing of the outer tube, frequent cleaning of any inner tube, good humidification and suction should prevent blockage from occurring. If suction and a change of inner tube fail to remove the obstruction (which is usually a large blob of mucus or a crust) the outer tube must be changed immediately. Occasionally even this is ineffective and emergency bronchoscopy is necessary to remove the obstruction. A spare tube, tapes and a tracheal dilator must always be at hand for an urgent tube change.

Displacement of the Tube

The tube can be displaced into the pretracheal tissues and it can come completely out of the stoma. This is most likely to occur if the tapes have not been tied correctly. The tracheostomy opening should be kept open with dilators. Summon help and insert the spare tube; if there are no dilators, spare tube, or help immediately available reinsert the same tube.

If a long tracheostomy tube is used, particularly in a low stoma, the end of the tube may enter the right main bronchus and prevent air entry into the left lung. Expansion of the unventilated side of the chest will be much reduced or absent and the patient may show signs of respiratory obstruction.

Surgical Emphysema

Surgical emphysema is caused by suturing the skin too tightly, so that air is directed into the tissues instead of leaking out around the tube. It is usually limited to the neck. If necessary the sutures can be released.

Dysphagia/Vomiting

If the tracheostomy tube is the wrong shape for the patient or is badly positioned it can cause pressure on the posterior tracheal wall and oesophagus. A different style of tube needs to be used.

Damage to the Tracheal Mucosa

Mucosal damage can be due to poor suction technique, a badly chosen or placed tube, or prolonged and excessive inflation of a cuff. Anterior wall ulceration can lead to fatal haemorrhage; posterior wall ulceration can produce a tracheo-oesophageal fistula. The long-term result of ulceration may be tracheal stenosis. Severe stenosis can occur if the cricoid cartilage or first tracheal ring has been damaged.

Infection

Wound and respiratory tract infections may occur, especially if aseptic techniques have not been practised during suction, stoma toilet and tube changing. Inadequate humidification and suction, which result in crust formation, predispose to pneumonia. It is important to remember that in bypassing the upper respiratory tract, tracheostomy removes most of the natural mechanisms available to protect the lower air passages. An infected tracheostomy wound needs at least as many aseptic changes of dressing and cleaning as any other infected wound.

Resuscitation of the Patient with a Tracheostomy

Mouth to mouth resuscitation is clearly inappropriate. An Ambu bag connected via corrugated tubing to a 15 mm connector (Fig. 26.5) which will fit onto a Portex or Shiley cuffed tracheostomy tube is necessary. As long as the cuff is inflated manual ventilation can be given.

If there is a plain tube *in situ*, and it is not possible to change this to a cuffed tube, then mouth to stoma ventilation can be given. The mouth and nose are sealed to prevent air leak by holding the chin up with the thumb to close the mouth whilst pinching the nose shut between the first and index fingers of the same hand. The mouth is then applied around the opening of the tracheostomy tube and ventilation given as for mouth-to-mouth resuscitation.

External cardiac massage should be given as for any other person requiring resuscitation.

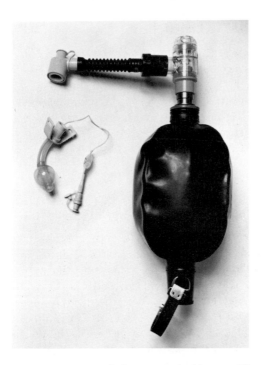

Fig. 26.5   An Ambu bag connected via corrugated tubing to a 15 mm connector. A Portex Profile tracheostomy tube with the cuff inflated is also illustrated.

Tracheostomy Tubes

Of the many different types of tracheostomy tubes available to cater for individual needs, silver and PVC are the most widely used materials; tubes made of duralite, stainless steel and silicone are also available. A tracheostomy tube is kept in position with tapes which are knotted at each side of the neck. When a patient has a tracheostomy there must be a spare tube of the same size and style, tapes and tracheal dilators at hand lest the tube fall out or need to be changed in an emergency. An open pair of tracheal dilators is shown in Fig. 26.6. The proximal end of a silver tracheostomy tube is equal in internal diameter to the distal end which lies in the trachea. In some PVC tubes the bore of the proximal end is standardized in size to enable it to be connected to anaesthetic or ventilating equipment, but the bore at the distal end varies according to the size of the tube.

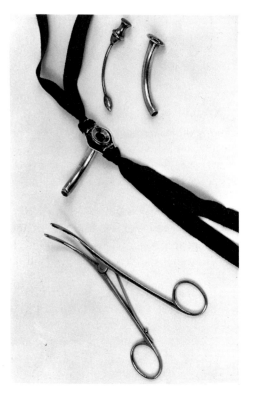

Fig. 26.6   A Negus tracheostomy tube with an inner tube in place. Also illustrated is the second inner tube, introducer and an open pair of tracheal dilators.

The size of the tube is noted on the flange. Most silver tubes have been graded in size according to the Charriere (French) gauge which refers to the external circumference of the tube in millimetres. British made PVC tubes are sized in mm according to the internal diameter (I/D). Most British tubes have both FG and mm sizes noted on the flange and packaging. Tubes made in North America, for example Shiley tubes, are not measured by these two methods but by numbers which can vary according to tube design. Ample literature with details of internal and external diameters is supplied with these tubes to enable one to choose the correct size.

Silver Tubes

Silver tubes are rigid, expensive and durable. Each set has an outer and inner tube, as well as an introducer (or obturator). The inner tube is slightly longer than the outer tube, so that any secretions or crusts which collect around the bottom of the tube come out when the inner tube is removed for cleaning, at least twice daily. The inner tube must be reinserted as soon as possible after cleaning; generally the outer tube need only be changed weekly. The introducer aids smooth insertion of the outer tube with a minimum of trauma; it must be removed as soon as the tube is inserted as it completely occludes the tube.

The parts of each silver tube set are not interchangeable, that is, they cannot be matched with the same part of another set of the same style and size, as they are not mass produced. If one part of a set is broken or lost then the remaining parts are no longer usable. However, some manufacturers will produce pairs of matching sets so that each patient has two outer and inner tubes and introducers which are interchangeable. Thus there can be one inner tube in position whilst the other is being cleaned and autoclaved if necessary.

Tubes can be cleaned by first being soaked in a solution, (e.g. sodium bicarbonate) which will loosen any mucus. The lumen of the tube should then be thoroughly cleaned under running water using a Magills or bottle brush of suitable size and used only for that patient. If the tube is too small to allow a brush to pass through, strips of 1.25 or 2.50 cm ribbon gauze can be pushed through the tube to ensure that the inside is clean. The tubes are

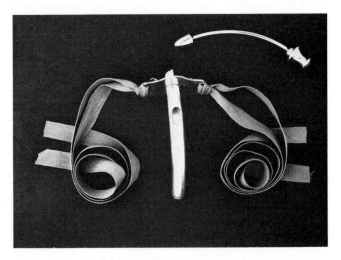

Fig. 26.7 A Chevalier Jackson's silver tracheostomy tube which has been fenestrated.

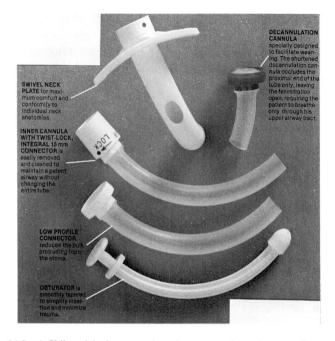

Fig. 26.8 A Shiley plain fenestrated tracheostomy tube and accessories.

sterilized by available methods. Tubes must always be dried thoroughly and stored dry rather than in a sterilizing fluid which can act as a culture medium for micro-organisms.

Silver tubes can be cleaned with household silver polish to remove tarnish marks. At home the patient can boil the tubes in a small saucepan, kept only for that purpose, before storing them dry.

The Negus silver tracheostomy tube set (Fig. 26.6) has one outer tube, an introducer and two inner tubes. One inner tube is plain, the other has a silver speaking valve flap which closes during expiration allowing air to pass through the larynx and the patient to speak.

The Chevalier Jackson set (Fig. 26.7) has only one inner tube; this can be 'locked' into place removing the possibility of its coming out during a bout of coughing. Another feature of the inner tube is that it has a small wing at each side which helps removal and insertion. This set has no valved inner tube to enable the patient to speak, but De Santi valves are available for this purpose.

The Chevalier Jackson tube illustrated (p. 243) is fenestrated; this allows air to pass through the larynx so that the patient can speak by putting his finger over the tube.

PVC Tubes

All PVC tubes are disposable. Whereas simple PVC tubes are quite cheap the more complex models are quite expensive in the long run when compared to the durable silver tubes. Although most are intended to be used only once, plain tubes can be re-used by the same patient if they are cleaned thoroughly. PVC tubes are much lighter than silver and some patients prefer them for this reason. When at body temperature PVC softens a little, which silver never does, and sometimes this makes them more comfortable to wear. PVC tubes are always used when radiotherapy is given to an area including the tracheostomy as when a metal is present in the area being treated tissue necrosis is likely to occur. PVC tubes may be either plain or cuffed.

PLAIN PVC TUBES

Plain PVC tubes can be used when an adult does not require assisted respiration. In a child, a sufficient seal in the trachea can be achieved without the use of a cuff, permitting intermittent positive pressure ventilation (IPPV). Plain tubes can also be used following laryngectomy.

Some Portex plain tracheostomy tubes do not have an inner tube or introducer. Good humidification and suction are essential to keep the lumen of the tube clean. The blue line on the tube is radio opaque.

The many features of the Shiley plain fenestrated tube are shown and explained in Fig. 26.8.

CUFFED PVC TUBES

Cuffed PVC tubes are used when IPPV is required—a properly inflated cuff will ensure that the gases being delivered will enter the lungs and not escape through the larynx. An inflated cuff will also prevent saliva, nasal secretions, regurgitated gastric contents and blood from entering the lower part of the respiratory tract. Low-volume, high-pressure cuffs are sometimes deflated for 2–10 minutes every hour to relieve pressure on the tracheal mucosa; it is doubtful, however, that the blood supply to the tracheal mucosa recovers sufficiently to reverse any ischaemic changes. When a cuffed tube is *in situ* it should be remembered that the cuff should only be inflated as necessary and deflated when possible. Inflation of the cuff should be just sufficient to create a seal between the cuff and the tracheal wall. There are pressure gauges available to monitor cuff pressure, which should be below 25 cm water. The volume of air in the cuff must always be recorded, as should the periods of time that it is kept inflated and deflated.

Before inserting a cuffed tube it is necessary to remove residual air from the cuff with a syringe. The pilot balloon will indicate whether the cuff is inflated or deflated when the tube is in position.

A Profile tube may also be employed. Like the Shiley cuffed tube, the Profile tube has a thin-walled low-pressure, high-volume cuff which minimizes the possibility of damage to the tracheal mucosa and does not need to be deflated intermittently.

RECURRENT LARYNGEAL NERVE PALSY

Adduction of the vocal cords and closure of the glottis is a relatively strong movement (because of this, intrathoracic pressure can be raised to the systolic blood pressure against the closed glottis) whereas abduction is a weak movement. The paralysed vocal cord lies in an adducted position and lacks tone; the quality of the voice changes and is weaker. The changes vary considerably from patient to patient; some can even sing in tune over a limited range while in others the paralysed cord may be a chance finding in a patient with no vocal symptoms. If both sides are paralysed the airway is severely restricted.

The laryngeal musculature is supplied by the recurrent laryngeal nerve which reaches the larynx from below, passing upwards between the trachea and oesophagus. On the right side it has looped around the subclavian artery but on the left it loops around the aorta and is vulnerable to disease within the chest. The left side is more commonly paralysed than the right.

Aetiology

In about 50% of the cases seen in the outpatient department, no identifiable cause is found and of these almost all recover spontaneously (generally within 6 months). Of the other 50% the commonest cause is from bronchial carcinoma and in the next largest group the paralysis is a consequence of thyroidectomy. Other causes are much less common and include carcinoma of the thyroid and of the oesophagus and involvement in the mediastinum by enlarged lymph nodes. Disease of the central nervous system, particularly motor neurone disease and also some cases of cerebro-vascular accidents affect the lower cranial nerves, producing cord paralysis and dysphagia. There is a large group in which the paralysis seems to follow a flu-like illness.

Treatment

If both cords are involved, a tracheostomy is required to restore an adequate airway. On a long term basis, a tracheostomy tube incorporating an expiratory valve will enable the patient to breathe via the tube but on expiration with closure of the valve, air is directed through the larynx as the cords are not tightly apposed. This flow of air can be used for phonation. Alternatively, an operation on the larynx to improve the airway can be carried out (e.g. Woodman's operation) though the bigger the airway, the poorer the speech quality.

For unilateral palsy, the quality of the voice may be improved by speech therapy so the patient learns to make the best use of the limited function. In appropriate cases the paralysed cord may be made more rigid by an injection of teflon paste; this can sometimes result in a good singing voice.

INFORMATION SOURCES

Portex Limited,
Hythe,
Kent.

Shiley Limited,
42 Thames Street,
Windsor,
Berkshire.

27 Tumours of the Head and Neck and their Treatment

GENERAL PRINCIPLES

In Britain malignant tumours of the head and neck form only a small proportion (about 7%) of malignant disease; elsewhere the incidence and site may be peculiar to that part of the world (e.g. Burkitt's lymphoma of central Africa and the high incidence of carcinoma of the nasopharynx among the Chinese).

The particular problems of malignant disease in this site include obstruction to air and food passages and disfigurement.

These tumours may usually be visualized on examination and are often palpable, thus their progress can be readily assessed. Where there is bone destruction X-rays and more recently Nuclear Magnetic Resonance Imaging (MRI), are invaluable both to determine the extent of the tumour and in the planning of treatment. MRI is a technique which displays internal soft tissues and which has been increasingly used in recent years (though it is very expensive). It depends on the effect of an intense magnetic field on molecules of water which then tend to become orientated in a particular way depending on their electrical charge. This property is called Nuclear Magnetic Resonance. An example of the quality of detail obtained is shown in Fig. 27.1; it is of particular value in ENT in displaying tumours of the head and neck. It does not involve the use of X-rays. The CT scan and the use of fibreoptic endoscopy may supplement this information.

Untreated these diseases frequently prove fatal while the disease is still localized above the clavicles. There may be spread to adjacent lymph nodes (even into the mediastinum) but spread to lungs, liver and elsewhere is rare. This has encouraged attempts to control the disease by surgical excision. Unfortunately even with extensive surgery, the prognosis is often poor; it is more related to the nature of the tumour and its precise site than to the extent of

248

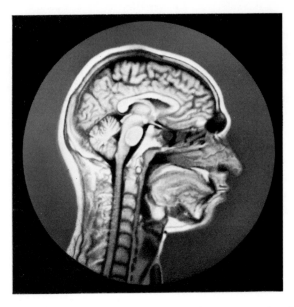

Fig. 27.1 MRI scan of the head and neck. MRI scan reproduced by kind permission of Queen's Square Imaging Centre, 8–11 Queen's Square, London, WC1N.

the excision. Such surgery is mutilating, but plastic surgery and prostheses will do much to restore function and contour. However, one must bear in mind that untreated the disease itself is often mutilating and noisome.

Many of the tumours are radiosensitive and a common plan of treatment is to give a course of radiotherapy and assess the response; surgery can be reserved for tumours not cured or which recur later. Alternatively primary surgery may be followed by radiotherapy to destroy any suspicious areas which may have been left at operation. A typical regime would be to give radiation daily during a 5 week period to a total dose of 5000 rad (1 rad = 0.01 Ey). A fit person may normally be treated as an outpatient.

The morbidity of X-ray therapy must not be underestimated. At the most trivial it abolishes mucus secretion producing dryness and hence discomfort in the air and food passages; at the other extreme it may induce so much oedema of the larynx for example, that a laryngectomy has to be performed.

More recently, chemotherapy with cytotoxic drugs has become widely used. Regimes to determine the best response from them are continually under trial. They may be used in conjunction with radiotherapy and/or surgery. Although expensive, if they are effective they would be particularly useful in those parts of the world where radiotherapy is not available.

CARCINOMA OF THE LARYNX

The commonest malignant tumour in (Western) ENT practice is carcinoma of the larynx. Almost all victims of this disease give a history of heavy cigarette smoking—it is rare in non-smokers. If the tumour is confined to the vocal cords it causes dysphonia and presents early. At this stage the cure rate with radiotherapy is 90%. Adverse features include loss of mobility of the cords, a site of origin either above or below the cords, spread to adjacent regions and lymph node involvement. Laryngectomy may be the initial treatment of choice (e.g. for a tumour which is considered incurable by radiotherapy). Alternatively excision may be reserved for tumours which fail to respond to radiotherapy or which recur later, or sometimes laryngectomy follows radiotherapy as a planned procedure, the theory being that the radiotherapy may arrest or reverse the spread of the disease so that subsequent excision is more likely to be complete. However, radiation devitalizes tissue, diminishes the blood supply and causes fibrosis and scarring; operating through an irradiated field is more difficult technically and more prone to give postoperative problems particularly fistulae, wound breakdown and major vessel erosion. This is now becoming less of a problem as with new techniques, the skin is subject to less radiation.

Pre-operative Care

The patient will be admitted to hospital several days before the operation for physical and psychological preparation. He will have already been in hospital for laryngoscopy and biopsy.

It is important to find out at an early stage how much knowledge and understanding the patient has of laryngectomy. Most people require several explanations as there is a large amount of information to assimilate. Simple line drawings can be helpful when explaining the effect of removing the larynx on the airway. Some hospitals have produced a small booklet containing a realistic account of the pre-operative, postoperative, and recovery periods. This is a useful supplement to verbal explanation and discussions, not a substitute. The whole family must be included and encouraged to ask questions.

Information about nasogastric tube feeding, intravenous infusion, dressings and drains and tracheal suction must be given. If it is known that a tube is to be in place in the end-tracheostome created at the time of surgery, then a description of the tube should be given. There is usually no reason why the patient cannot see and handle some of the equipment which will be used.

Patients will be mute for several weeks after surgery. A 'special nurse' should be in attendance for the first 24 hours and the patient reassured that he will not be left alone during this time. A call bell, pen and paper must be seen to be available before surgery. If the patient is illiterate non-verbal communication signs can be practised, picture card signs can be discussed and added to if necessary. If good relationships and communication can be established before surgery the patient can look forward to the postoperative period with more confidence.

The Role of Other Disciplines

The care before and after surgery is shared with the speech therapist, physiotherapist and medical social worker. Good communication between all disciplines is essential.

The speech therapist will want to form a relationship with the patient before surgery is performed. The therapist assesses how articulate the patient is and the extent of his vocabulary and gives explanations of how voice can be achieved following laryngectomy. At this stage some therapists like to introduce to the patient a person of similar age and circumstances who has had a laryngectomy and developed good oesophageal speech, but the wishes of the patient should always be taken into consideration.

Prior to surgery the patient will be taught deep breathing and leg exercises by the physiotherapist who will also explain the care the patient will receive for his altered airway during the recovery period. Anti-emboli stockings, to reduce the risk of deep vein thrombosis, may be worn during the pre-operative period and until the patient is mobile after surgery.

The majority of the patients and their families need the services of a social worker. The help that is given is not only financial but will also include emotional and psychological support, and possibly help with employment.

Physical Preparation

Physical preparation will include an ECG and a selection of blood tests and X-rays. Swabs of the nose and throat and specimens of sputum are taken for culture and sensitivity. Dental health is checked and any carious teeth removed.

The patient may be malnourished if dysphagia has been a problem in which case this should be corrected pre-operatively. A simple aperient and/or suppository is usually sufficient to ensure that the bowel is empty on the day of operation. Body hair between the chin and nipples should be removed. A man will also need a full face shave on the morning of the operation. A sedative or hypnotic may be required the night before surgery.

Breathing through a tracheostome for ever and being unable to speak for several weeks is a daunting prospect. Good pre-operative explanation and preparation play a major part in helping the patient make a satisfactory postoperative recovery.

Postoperative Care

Before the patient returns from the operating theatre all equipment necessary for the immediate postoperative period should be assembled and checked to ensure that it is in good working order. The equipment is the same as for tracheostomy, except that tracheal dilators are not essential.

The patient will return in his own bed. He will be nursed in a semi-recumbent position at first then gradually helped into an upright position well supported with pillows. This position improves respiration and aids wound drainage. The neck should be kept flexed to avoid tension on the suture lines.

Patients can usually sit out of bed and take a few steps the day following surgery; this is increased as they feel able to spend longer periods out of bed. Initially, the vital signs are recorded at half hourly intervals then gradually reduced as the condition improves.

A nasogastric feeding tube will be *in situ*, and will require aspiration at intervals of 1–4 hours. It is important to prevent vomiting as this may damage the pharyngeal suture line. Feeding is commenced on the first or second postoperative day. The tube remains for about 10 days, possibly longer if radiotherapy has been given, to allow the pharyngeal repair to heal. A check for fistula formation can be made before the tube is removed (see Chapter 24). Should the nasogastric tube come out it should not be re-inserted by a nurse lest the pharyngeal repair be damaged. Most surgeons would prefer the patient to have parenteral feeding rather than risk damage by reinserting a feeding tube. If patients show an interest they can be taught how to give their own bolus feeds. Regular oral hygiene is essential; morning coffee and afternoon tea can be given as a 'mouthwash' to most patients. The inability to hold the breath and increase intrathoracic and abdominal pressures during defaecation can cause constipation. This is usually remedied by using a simple aperient, or when food is being taken by mouth, the fibre content in the diet increased.

The wound is usually drained with either suction or corrugated drains. Drainage normally ceases within 4 days and must be observed for saliva which would indicate fistula formation. If a pressure dressing is applied it should remain for 24–48 hours. It should be possible to slip a finger down between the back of the neck and bandage to ensure that it is not too tight. Too tight a bandage can restrict blood flow and the patient becomes cyanosed from the bandage upwards, while the other extremities are pink and well oxygenated. In this situation the bandage must be cut and another bandage applied on top. If the wound is satisfactory when the pressure bandage is removed, it can either be left exposed or a light gauze dressing or spray-on dressing can be applied. Wound sutures are removed 7–10 days after surgery.

The period following laryngectomy has some problems in common with tracheostomy, for example loss of cough and humidification. Nursing actions to reduce these are described in Chapter 25. Initially tracheal secretions are profuse and tracheal suction will be required. Generally, secretions gradually lessen in amount and by the time patients are ready to go home they are able to exporate all of their secretions. However, some patients will require the use of a suction machine at home. Before such patients go home they, and whenever possible a member of their families, must be taught how to perform tracheal suction. The need for a clean technique needs to be stressed. Laryngectomy results in a permanent alteration to the respiratory tract (Fig.

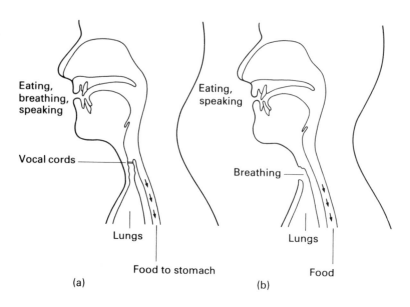

Fig. 27.2   (a) Before laryngectomy; (b) after laryngectomy.

27.2). There are various tubes (Fig. 27.3 and 27.4) that can be used in the end-tracheostome created at the time of surgery. The tube or button is changed once or twice daily. There is no need for tracheal dilators to be at hand unless there is a large amount of oedema, or a skin flap around the stoma. A tube can safely be changed by one nurse as, unlike tracheostomy, the danger of sudden closure of the opening does not exist. The stoma needs to be cleaned thoroughly each time the tube is changed. Crusts should be removed using Tilley's forceps. When no tube is *in situ* the stoma still needs to be cleaned several times daily, and observations for stenosis made. The stoma is to remain for life so the patient needs to be taught the care that is necessary to keep it clean. Initially the patient is encouraged to observe the nurse in a mirror and is then supervised and given support whilst doing his own care. Early involvement will help the patient to come to terms with his altered body.

Communication by writing is time consuming, tiring and frustrating, and it is little wonder that some patients get depressed and withdrawn following surgery. The nurse must show understanding when caring for these patients as the problems they encounter are

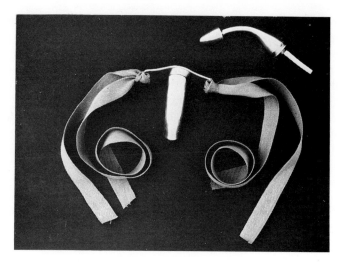

Fig. 27.3 The Colledge silver laryngectomy tube with introducer.

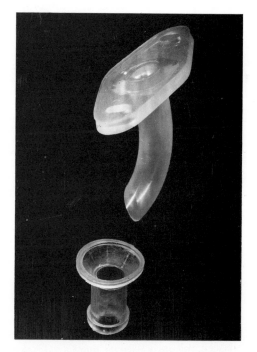

Fig. 27.4 The Shah silastic laryngectomy tube and a stoma button.

many, particularly when communication is difficult. Some nurses achieve a considerable skill in lip reading. Once the nasogastric tube is removed and oral feeding is established speech therapy can begin and will continue for several months. Initial efforts at voice production can be frustrating and embarrassing and this may discourage and depress the patient. The nurse should allow the patient time and avoid the temptation to finish words or sentences. If the patient says five words and only three are understood, do not ask the patient to repeat the understood words; ask him to repeat only what has not been understood, otherwise the patient may become discouraged and return to pen and paper to 'save the nurses' time'.

It is estimated that 60% of patients achieve oesophageal voice. There are mechanical aids available both for those unable to

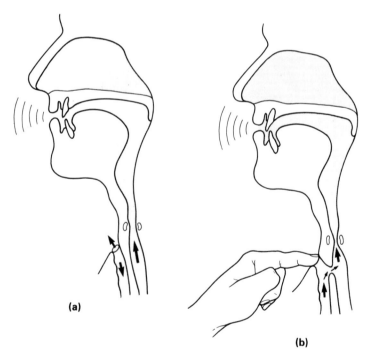

Fig. 27.5 Differences between oesophageal and fistula voice production. (a) Air is forced upwards from the oesophagus, respiration is independent; (b) manual occlusion of the stoma diverts air through the fistula into the oesophagus during expiration.

produce oesophageal voice and for the patient who has a fistula or wound breakdown (which will prevent speech therapy being commenced until healing is complete). There is also a place for these to aid communication when the patient first goes home. In suitable patients, by surgically creating a fistula between trachea and oesophagus, expired air can be used for voice production. Figure 27.5 illustrates the difference between oesophageal and fistula voice production. The Staffieri primary neoglottic technique includes reconstruction at the time of laryngectomy, and allows voice to be achieved at an earlier stage. Alternatively a Blom Singer or a Panje valve may be inserted after laryngectomy. However, problems such as leakage of saliva and fluid through the fistula into the trachea can occur.

Laryngectomy can result in the loss of several things that one usually takes for granted. The sound of laughter can no longer be made and singing is denied to the majority. The sense of smell can be affected as air is no longer drawn through the nasal cavity. Laryngectomy patients can feel that by losing their original voice they have lost a large part of their personality. The male voice and larynx undergo considerable change at puberty and many men associate masculinity with the larynx and the voice. In our society the accepted norm for a female is a voice with a much higher, but softer, pitch than the rather harsh low pitched sound which is produced from the upper oesophagus. Until recently swimming was not possible, however, swimming aids are now available but medical advice and supervision must be sought. As long as the stoma is protected showers can be taken. A hot steaming bath can be a useful form of humidification at home.

Rehabilitation is an ongoing process; as discharge approaches the patient can be introduced to various aids. The box illustrated in Fig. 27.6 contains a selection of useful items (and information on where they can be obtained) which the patients and their family can see, handle and discuss.

Should resuscitation be required at any stage mouth to stoma ventilation will need to be given until a cuffed tracheostomy tube can be inserted and connected to an Ambu bag (Chapter 26, Fig. 26.5).

Many hospitals have a Laryngectomy Club which is run by staff involved in laryngectomy. These clubs are of social and therapeutic value to patients and families. The National Association of Laryngectomee Clubs organizes discussions and seminars for all

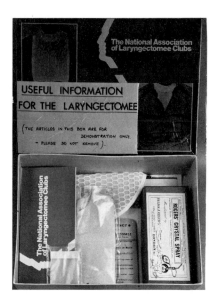

Fig. 27.6 A box containing information leaflets and useful appliances such as stoma protectors can be assembled and used when discussing self care and preparing the laryngectomee for discharge.

disciplines involved in laryngectomy care as well as giving much advice and support to those who have had a laryngectomy.

CARCINOMA OF THE HYPOPHARYNX

Carcinoma of the post cricoid region and of the pyriform fossae has a poor prognosis as it presents late and spreads early both locally and to regional lymph nodes. These patients are not in good general condition because of dysphagia. Unfortunately these tumours often respond poorly to radiotherapy. Surgery involves excision of larynx and pharynx with the fashioning of an end tracheostome and the construction of a new food passage. This may be achieved by one of several ways, for example, by a 'pull up' operation in which the oesophagus is removed and the stomach is brought up and joined to the pharynx, or the colon may be used as a graft in a similar way, or it may be by local skin flaps. In the case of small tumours there may be sufficient healthy pharyngeal mucosa spare to allow primary closure.

Pre-operative Care

Pharyngo-laryngo-oesophagectomy with gastric anastomosis includes total thyroidectomy and parathyroidectomies. The number of structures removed and the subsequent alterations to the patient's anatomy and physiology are difficult enough for professionals to immediately appreciate and understand, and this must be remembered when explanations are being given to the patient and his family.

Physical Preparation

This is a major surgical procedure that requires a number of pre-operative investigations. A 3 day bowel preparation and cleansing programme is carried out in case it is necessary to use colon to replace oesophagus (if it should prove impossible to mobilize the stomach). Body hair between chin and pubic area is removed in preparation for the surgery.

The patient is likely to be malnourished owing to dysphagia and steps to correct this should be taken before surgery. As the patient is likely to remain in bed for several days anti-emboli stockings are worn from the day before surgery until full mobility is achieved.

Psychological Preparation

Psychological preparation is very important and is similar to that described prior to laryngectomy. It is wise to inform the family as well as the patient about the large number of attachments for example, drains, cardiac monitor, that are going to be used and that visits should be limited during the immediate postoperative period.

The social worker, speech therapist and physiotherapist are involved in the care from an early stage. An ENT surgeon performs the neck and throat surgery, the abdominal part of the operation being carried out by a general surgeon.

Postoperative Care

The patient will need a special nurse for at least the first 48 hours. Figure 27.7 shows the various drains etc. that are likely to be in position immediately after surgery.

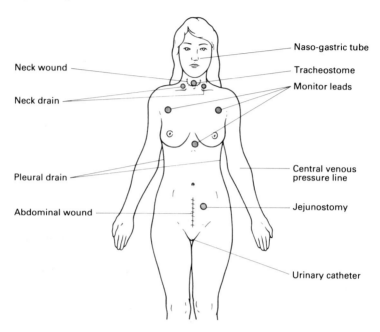

Fig. 27.7   Pharyngo-laryngo oesophagectomy, with gastric anastomies. Illustration shows the position of the various drains and appliances.

The presence of an end-tracheostome creates the same problems as in total laryngectomy. However, owing to the pain caused by the abdominal wound, respiratory movements and coughing are difficult, so deep tracheal suction using angled catheters is necessary. Humidified oxygen is likely to be required for at least the first day. The care of the neck wounds and drains follows the same pattern as laryngectomy.

If a nasogastric tube is *in situ* it is either left on free drainage or aspirated every hour to keep the stomach empty, as vomiting jeopardizes the anastomosis. When bowel movements return feeding is commenced via the jejunostomy. This may cause considerable diarrhoea at first, and accurate fluid balance records must be maintained. Small amounts of fluid and semi-solids are usually given by mouth after about 5 days, but it is likely to be at least 2 weeks before an adequate diet can be taken by mouth and the jejunostomy closed. The skin around the jejunostomy can become very excoriated from intestinal secretions unless it is protected.

A urinary catheter is in position for the first 2 days at least and during this time regular catheter toilet using an aseptic technique is essential. Initially, urinary output and specific gravity is recorded hourly to assess renal function which can be impaired owing to ischaemia if the patient is, or has been, hypovolaemic (or shocked).

The patient is unlikely to be able to get out of bed before the second postoperative day, and is likely to be underweight and debilitated—regular, frequent changes of position are essential if pressure sores are to be avoided and comfort maintained.

By the third postoperative day the patient is generally beginning to feel better and some of the drains, tubes, etc., will have been removed. (The two pleural drains, which are attached to underwater-seal drainage bottles are, on average, removed after 3 days.) However, the inability to communicate can be felt more deeply now and the patient's emotional needs increase. When the stomach is attached to the base of the tongue, pseudovoice can be achieved earlier than following laryngectomy; however, the quality of the voice is usually poorer making communication difficult.

Once oral feeding is established and there is no problem with regurgitation of stomach contents into the mouth the patient can lie flat in bed rather than stay in a sitting up position. A pyloroplasty and vagotomy are performed (when the stomach is mobilized) to aid gastric emptying; however, the patient is never going to be able to indulge in a large meal and small frequent meals will be the rule. Many patients have had marked dysphagia prior to surgery and this will be a vast improvement for them.

There will be frequent follow up and speech therapy sessions after the patient is discharged. This is a relatively rare operation and most nurses in the community would welcome the chance to visit the patient in hospital and discuss his care with the hospital nurses before the patient goes home. The patient's family should feel able to telephone the hospital should they experience problems.

CARCINOMA OF THE PARANASAL SINUSES

Carcinoma of the maxillary and ethmoid sinuses is treated by chemotherapy, radiotherapy and/or surgical excision.

Pre-operative Care

Maxillectomy involves removal of the maxilla which includes the hard palate and the orbital floor; occasionally even the orbital contents are removed and the patient must be prepared for this. Physical and psychological preparation is similar to that required prior to other head and neck surgery. No local skin preparation is necessary. The eyebrows are not removed as the hair tends to regrow in a very irregular fashion. The care is shared with an oral surgeon. The patient will need to visit the oral surgery prosthetic department to have a dental plate prepared or an existing plate modified.

This will be a very anxious time for the patient and his family, and a great deal of reassurance will be needed along with several explanations of what maxillectomy entails.

Postoperative Care

When the patient is able he is gradually sat up in bed. Most patients are well enough to sit out of bed for short periods the day following surgery. Vital signs are taken at intervals consistent with individual needs.

Regular thorough oral hygiene is essential and may be needed every hour at first. Gentle irrigation is usually effective until the patient is able to rinse out his own mouth. Any remaining teeth can be cleaned with a small toothbrush.

A large pack (usually impregnated with Whitehead's varnish) will be in the cavity created by the removal of the maxilla for approximately 7 days. The pack is kept in place by a dental plate which is not removed for cleaning as long as the pack is *in situ*. Following removal of the pack the plate can, and must, be removed several times a day and cleaned with toothpaste and a toothbrush under running water. As soon as possible patients are taught how to do this for themselves. A permanent plate with an attached obturator, to give shape to the cheek, will be made when the cavity has healed and any oedema has subsided; however, by this time the patient has usually been discharged from hospital.

It may be necessary to irrigate the cavity with a solution of warm saline, 1% sodium bicarbonate or hydrogen peroxide 10 vol to remove debris after the pack has been removed. A Higginson's or plastic syringe with a catheter attached can be used. After being given an explanation the patient is seated in a comfortable upright position with clothing protected. The return fluid is collected in a receiver which can be held by the patient under his chin. Irrigation continues until the return fluid is clean. Any crusts in the cavity are left undisturbed unless the surgeon requests their removal, in which case the nurse must inspect the cavity thoroughly with a head mirror and use Tilley's nasal forceps to remove the crusts.

The suture line which extends from the middle of the lip, up the side of the nose and across the upper cheek in a skin crease under the lower eyelid, is left exposed. If the eyeball has been removed a pressure dressing is applied to this area in theatre and remains for approximately 1 day.

This area can then be kept covered with an eyepad until a prosthesis (an artificial eye and eyelids attached to a pair of spectacles) is made. Facial sutures are removed about a week after surgery.

An intravenous infusion is only required for 1–2 days; by this time the patient can usually manage an adequate oral intake. The patient may experience some problems with drinking and eating. The mouth is tender and some degree of trismus will be present. Some patients find a straw useful; others prefer to use a spouted feeding cup which allows the tongue to control the flow of fluid. Solid food must be soft as chewing is difficult. It can take the patient quite a long time to eat an adequate quantity of any meal offered, so small amounts need to be offered frequently to prevent the food getting cold and the patient tired and disheartened. Nutritional supplements, such as Clinifeed or Complan, are valuable additions.

Articulation may be difficult, especially if the plate is at all loose. Speech can sound a little slurred, so the nurse should look and listen carefully when the patient is speaking.

Most patients are ready for discharge a few days after the pack is removed. The patient must be able to remove, clean and reinsert the dental plate before going home. Follow-up by oral and ENT surgeons is necessary. The oral surgery staff will teach the patient the care of the final obturator when it is made.

CRANIOFACIAL RESECTION

Craniofacial resection is undertaken via an extended lateral rhinotomy incision. Exposure of the floor of the anterior cranial

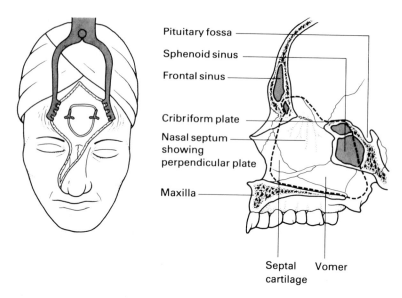

Pituitary fossa

Sphenoid sinus

Frontal sinus

Cribriform plate

Nasal septum
showing
perpendicular plate

Maxilla

Septal   Vomer
cartilage

Fig. 27.8 Craniofacial resection. Extent of the resection which may be undertaken. Reproduced by kind permission of *Nursing* magazine.

fossa to determine the operability of the tumour is achieved by a frontal craniotomy (Fig. 27.8).

Structures which can be removed include the maxilla, ethmoid bone (with cribriform and perpendicular plates), part of the sphenoid bone, the nasal septum and the orbit with its contents. The nasal fossae and sinuses are concerted into one cavity by the procedure.

Pre-operative Care

Both the patient and his family need a great deal of support pre-operatively. A thorough explanation of the procedure and subsequent events is essential, as well as all the other aspects of psychological and physical preparation necessary before surgery, including the services of a social worker.

Depilation of the donor skin graft area (usually the thigh), is required.

Postoperative Care

In order to maintain intracranial pressure the patient is nursed in a supine position, with one or two pillows, for the first 5 days after surgery. Careful attention is given to the prevention of pressure sores and potential circulatory and respiratory problems. After this period gradual mobilization is started. Some patients may find this enforced inactivity very boring and frustrating. Visitors and the media can help prevent boredom but should be limited to allow the patient adequate rest.

Initial neurological and vital signs are recorded at frequent intervals as cerebral oedema can occur, and may cause a cerebro-vascular accident or grand mal seizure. Prophylactic Phenytoin or Phenobarbitone can be given to suppress cerebral irritation and reduce the likelihood of seizures. Observations are gradually reduced according to the patient's condition.

Fluids will be given by an intravenous infusion until the patient is able to take an adequate diet by mouth; this is usually 24–48 hours. Whilst the patient is on bed rest assistance with fluids and meals is necessary. The patient may benefit from an antacid to reduce gastric acid regurgitation during this time.

A self retaining urinary catheter is in position for the first few days to enable a continuous, accurate fluid balance to be calculated (diabetes insipidus is a possible complication). It may be left in position until the patient is mobile if problems in micturition are anticipated owing to the patient having to remain on total bed rest. Whilst the catheter is in position regular catheter care using an aseptic technique is performed.

A pack, usually ribbon gauze impregnated with Whitehead's varnish, is inserted into the cavity created by the removal of the tumour and structures involved. The pack is removed, under a general anaesthetic 10–14 days after surgery. During this time antibiotic therapy is in progress. Observations for cerebrospinal fluid rhinorrhoea need to be made. The presence of the pack results in constant mouth breathing so frequent oral care is essential.

For approximately 2 days following surgery a pressure dressing is in position around the forehead and over the orbit on the affected side. Eye care may be necessary depending on the amount of soft tissue swelling. Following removal of this dressing the suture line can be left exposed. Sutures are removed approximately 6 days after surgery. If an eye has been removed the patient will appreciate an eye pad to cover the defect until a prosthesis can be made. The donor skin graft area on the thigh is usually covered with an op-site dressing which is, whenever possible, left undisturbed until the area has healed; this technique dramatically reduces postoperative pain from the donor site.

Craniofacial resection is an extensive surgical procedure yet the pain experienced by the patient following removal of the tumour is often less than before surgery, and one of the milder analgesics is usually sufficient. Strong narcotics are avoided during the immediate postoperative period as they can mask changes in the neurological and vital signs.

The patient is ready to go home fairly soon after the pack is removed. If nasal sniffs or douches are necessary to remove crusts the patient will need to be taught this procedure before discharge (see p. 151). Follow-up appointments are essential.

Throughout their stay in hospital patients and their families will need much reassurance and support from all involved. Care and support may need to be continued by the Community Nursing Services following discharge.

CARCINOMA OF THE MOUTH

Carcinoma of the anterior part of the tongue may do well with radiotherapy but the more posterior the site, the worse the prognosis: carcinoma here and elsewhere in the mouth is generally treated with radiotherapy followed by surgery for residual disease. Surgery may well need to be extensive, with removal of much of the mandible and reconstruction of the mouth. Tumours in these areas are prone to have multifocal origin, and successful treatment of one tumour may well be followed by the appearance of another. These patients need careful follow up so that recurrence can be detected early.

Notwithstanding what has been said above, the management has to be geared to the individual with due consideration of morale, outlook, general condition and expectations. The social background and the attitudes of the patient and of those who will be supporting him must also be taken into account. The patient's approach to being mutilated and his need to learn a new method of speech or communication are all important considerations.

Pre-operative Care

The Commando procedure consists of a 'COMbined Mandibulectomy And Neck Dissection Operation'. The subsequent defect in the mouth can be repaired with either a myocutaneous or forehead flap. A temporary tracheostomy is performed at the same time. The patient cannot be fed by mouth for several weeks following surgery; a gastrostomy may have been performed already in order to correct any pre-operative malnutrition and for postoperative feeding purposes.

The patient and his family will require several thorough explanations. This is a very disfiguring operation and a great deal of psychological care and support is necessary. The services of the physiotherapist, social worker and speech therapist are required before and after surgery. Many physical examinations are carried out before the operation and it is important to make sure that the patient has adequate opportunities to ask questions and to rest during this time.

If a forehead flap is to be used for repair then a low hairline or bushy sideburns should be removed. Chest hair should be removed if a myocutaneous flap is to be raised from this area. The site of the flap used to repair the oral cavity defect is covered with a split skin graft (SSG) from the thigh; therefore the thigh also needs to be free from hair.

Postoperative Care

At first the patient is nursed in a semi-recumbent posture and frequent vital sign recordings are taken. As his condition improves he is gradually sat up, remembering that his head and neck must be kept well supported at all times. Mobilization can normally commence the day after surgery.

Initially a cuffed tracheostomy tube is necessary to protect the lower respiratory tract but as soon as the patient can swallow saliva and cough, a plain tube is used. The tracheostomy will remain until the postoperative swelling has subsided and no further surgery is planned. The patient may still have marked communication problems following closure of the tracheostomy as articulation is going to be difficult. Detailed descriptions of tracheostomy problems and care are described in Chapter 26.

Mouth care is of paramount importance and may be required every hour at first. Each time this is done the repair must be checked for any alteration in colour and gaping or sign of infection in the suture line. Gentle irrigation using a disposable Kwill and syringe can be effective in keeping the mouth clean, and patients can, in time, do this themselves. When hydrogen peroxide is used it should be followed by water or saline to ensure that all debris has been removed. If suction is used to remove secretions or cleansing fluids from the mouth, then great care must be taken and the pressure kept low lest the graft be damaged.

The intravenous infusion is discontinued once the patient is tolerating an adequate amount via the nasogastric or gastrostomy route. Most patients can tolerate small amounts by the tube on the first day and feeding is usually well established by the second day. Oral feeding is not likely to start for 3–4 weeks. Care of the area around the feeding tube is important if excoriation of the skin is to be avoided.

If a forehead flap has been used, a pressure dressing is usually applied in theatre, to the forehead and remains for 48 hours. Following removal of this dressing the SSG (taken from the thigh) is applied on the ward to the forehead. This graft is then either redressed and left untouched for about a week or left exposed. If left exposed it is necessary to gently roll sterile cotton wool dressed applicators over the area several times daily to prevent small pockets of serous fluid collecting under the graft. Once the forehead flap has 'taken' in the mouth the flap is divided and the part not involved in filling in the defect is swung upwards and replaced on the forehead. If a myocutaneous flap has been used from the chest, a drain will be *in situ* for approximately 3 days. The chest wound is usually closed primarily and the sutures removed 10 days later; alternatively a SSG is used to cover the site of a myocutaneous flap, in which case the area will require the same care as that described for the forehead.

The donor area on the thigh is often covered with an op-site dressing which is left undisturbed until healing is complete (approximately 10 days). This area may well be the greatest source of pain and discomfort for the patient.

There will be at least one drain in the neck for several days. When the dissection is performed on the left side there is small risk of accidently damaging the thoracic duct, causing chyle (milky white, fatty fluid) to leak out of the lymphatic channel into the tissues. In such instances drainage must always be examined for chyle. Some surgeons prefer to immobilize the patient's shoulder on the operated side following neck dissection using a triangular bandage sling.

The patient is likely to be in hospital for at least 4 weeks. Once the area has healed the speech therapist may be able to help the patient overcome articulation difficulties. Chewing and swallowing may be difficult at first until the patient adjusts to the limitations imposed by such a large resection. This is a mutilating and disfiguring operation performed on a part of the body which cannot be hidden and the need for continuing care and support for the patient and his family cannot be over-emphasized.

Radiotherapy Nursing Care

The object of radiation therapy is to kill or damage the rapidly dividing tumour cells whilst sparing the normal cells on which the healing process depends.

The treatment lasts 5–7 weeks and the patient and his family are going to need support throughout this time. The majority of patients will be treated as outpatients.

General effects of radiotherapy include anorexia and nausea which can make it difficult for diet that is adequate in calories and nutrients to be taken. This is made worse by the loss of saliva, oral mucositis, pharyngitis and dysphagia depending on the treatment site. The patient, and his family, will need advice on dietary requirements and the use of supplements, such as Build-Up. The mouth can be very tender so spirits, spicy food and tobacco should be avoided. Mucaine or Aspirin gargles can be helpful in relieving discomfort and making swallowing easier. Distortion or loss of taste accompany a dry mouth; artificial saliva can make the mouth feel more comfortable and moist. Occasionally oral mucositis and pharyngitis can be severe enough to warrant hospitalization. The pain and discomfort experienced can result in a very distressed, malnourished and dehydrated patient who requires feeding by nasogastric tube or an intravenous infusion until the reaction has subsided.

The loss of saliva also makes the mouth more susceptible to infection, including candidiasis, so high standards in oral care must be maintained. Antiseptic mouthwashes can be an effective part of this care. It may be a year or more before salivary flow returns.

The skin can present problems for the patient. Most radiotherapists allow warm water to be used for washing as long as nothing is added to the water, and the treatment area is gently patted dry and not rubbed. Only prescribed medications should be used on the skin. Preparations containing zinc e.g. soap and cosmetics, are not used. The treatment area should be protected from sunlight and strong winds as these increase any skin reaction. Erythema will occur during treatment in most people. Radiotherapy has an effect on the skin similar to strong sunlight—the area first goes red, then dry, with moist desquamation following if over exposure or hypersensitivity occur. If a severe skin reaction does occur the radiotherapy is temporarily discontinued and the area treated, usually with steroid preparations, until the skin is healthy enough to allow radiotherapy to recommence. Men are advised to use an electric razor, this not only avoids wetting the area and using soap, but avoids the risk of skin abrasions at a time when healing is delayed and risk of infection increased.

Alopecia may occur, either at the site of entry or exit of the beam of radiation. If this is causing embarrassment a wig may be worn.

If there is a reduction in tears, eye bathing and the installation of soothing drops, for example artificial tear drops, can help relieve discomfort. The risk of conjunctivitis is increased by the absence of tears with their antiseptic and cleansing actions and antibiotic eye drops, with ointment at night, may be necessary.

When the larynx is being treated, voice rest is advised. It should be explained to the patient that this includes whispering. Oedema of the larynx causing stridor can occur making hospitalization, and possibly tracheostomy, necessary.

INFORMATION SOURCES

National Society for Cancer Relief,
Anchor House,
Britten Street,
London, SW3.

National Association of Laryngectomee Clubs,
4th Floor,
39 Eccleston Square,
London, SW1V 1PB.

Aid for Children with Tracheostomies,
A. Goadby,
8 Hampton Close,
Wigston Magna,
Leicester, LE8 1XD.

Let's Face It (A support network for the facially disfigured.)
Mrs C. Piff,
10 Wood End,
Crowthorn,
Berkshire.

28 Drugs in ENT

Ideally drugs should be effective, free from side-effects, cheap, simple in composition and easy to administer. They may be given topically or systematically: topical administration is particularly appropriate in ENT work because disease is localized and there is ready access to affected skin and mucosal surfaces.

NOSE

Topical Drugs

Topical administration may be by drops, spray or cream. Cream can be applied with the tip of a clean finger into the nasal vestibule. Naseptin cream (containing chlorhexidine and neomycin) is commonly used for vestibulitis or for crusting in the vestibule.

The use of liquid preparations in the form of drops is traditional, but an effective spray can nowadays be easily delivered by a 'squeezy' plastic container: a more finely dispersed (aerosol) mist can be delivered from a pressurized container or nebulizer in metred doses.

Vasoconstrictor Preparations

Sympathomimetic drugs constrict the arterioles in the nasal lining and increase the airway. Ephedrine 1% (or 0.5% in infants) is commonly prescribed. This will shrink the mucosa within a few minutes and the effect will last for a few hours. It is thus of value in the infant with URTI who is finding it difficult to suckle or feed because of the impaired airway: in the adult who is subject to otic barotrauma it is of value on aircraft journeys.

Popular and more powerful drugs are available (e.g. xylometazoline, oxymetazoline) and some without prescription. These have a more profound and prolonged effect but after several hours the effect wears off and the lining swells again (rebound). This may occur with ephedrine drops, but to a lesser extent. With the return of symptoms the patient takes another dose and the process is repeated. If, in this way, use is prolonged, there is gradually less response to the drug and finally a condition of rhinitis medicamentosa is produced in which the mucosa remains swollen and red (see p. 148). These drugs also inhibit the activity of the cilia in the nose. Because they have a sympathomimetic action, side effects include tachycardia; in particular they should not be given to patients concurrently taking mono-amine-oxidase inhibitors (a commonly used antidepressant) as the cardiovascular effects may well be accentuated. Similarly, caution may be advised in prescribing drugs for known hypertensive patients. More dilute solutions are available for paediatric use. Commonly such medicine is supplied in a small bottle incorporating a dropper in the cap: this is convenient but the contents of the bottle are at risk of being contaminated with nasal secretion carried on the dropper. The patient should not share his bottle with the family and should discard it when the course of treatment is complete. This problem does not occur when individual dose sachets are used (oxymetazoline is supplied in this form as *Iliadin-Mini*) which also prevents overdosage.

If the patient uses a spray when the nose is completely blocked, the drug is merely deposited on the anterior end of the inferior turbinate. This not only may be ineffective but it also leads to the anterior part of the nose becoming dry and sore, possibly with crusting or bleeding. In this situation, drops which can trickle past the obstruction, may be more effective than sprays.

Drugs Used in Rhinitis

For the patient suffering from a seasonal or perennial rhinitis, treatment is likely to be prolonged and drugs with a different action are more suitable. Cromoglycate is said to inhibit the release from sensitized cells (mast cells) of chemicals causing the allergic reaction but is thought to partially anaesthetize the mucosa. However it should be given prophylactically before symptoms develop. It is available in drops and sprays, nebulizers and as a fine powder (in spincaps).

Beclamethasone is available in similar forms; this anti-inflammatory steroid is effective but costly. Any systemic absorption is negligible. It seems to inhibit the recurrence of nasal polypi.

Simple sniffing of salt solution from the palm of the hand is helpful for patients troubled by crusting or secretions.

Cocaine

In the examination of the nose and for minor outpatient procedures (e.g. antral lavage, cautery, nasal polypectomy) it is common in Britain to use a cocaine spray; a mixture of 10% cocaine with an equal quantity of 1:1000 adrenaline is popular. The adrenaline deteriorates on exposure to light and these solutions should preferably be freshly prepared or kept in the dark. This preparation shrinks the nasal lining giving a better view and access; it produces vasoconstriction, reducing bleeding (thus being of value in epistaxis) and it also has a marked local anaesthetic action. Patients may experience troublesome sneezing and irritation of the nose on the way home as its effect wears off. It can also be applied on a pledget of cotton wool, but should be used sparingly, the pledget being wrung out. Toxic effects are convulsions but restlessness, tachycardia and elevation of blood pressure are earlier signs and if indicated, are treated by sedation e.g. by diazepam. A safer local anaesthetic for topical application is a 4% solution of lignocaine, but this does not have the vasoconstrictive effect.

Similarly cetacaine spray is available in a pressurized container and may be used to anaesthetize the pharynx if the patient is unable to suppress the gag reflex when the larynx or nasopharynx is examined with a mirror.

Inhalations

Steam inhalations have been used over the centuries, but the essential value of this treatment is that water is deposited on the mucosal surfaces: there is little evidence that the various additives (menthol, pine etc.) have any extra value except that they may have a pleasant smell, a relief to the patient with a reduced sense of smell.

Systemic Drugs

The most commonly prescribed systemic drugs for nasal conditions are antihistamines such as chlorpheniramine (Piriton) and promethazine (Phenergan), or drugs which incorporate antihistamines. These neutralize the histamine released as part of the allergic response and are thus of particular value in hay fever. They also have a parasympatholytic (atropine like) effect which makes them of value in those cases of intrinsic rhinitis where an allergen cannot be incriminated. Probably all the antihistamines have some sedative action, more marked with some (e.g. Phenergan, which is a useful hypnotic especially in children) than with others (e.g. mebhydrolin, Fabahistin, Ferferadine). For patients who are troubled by nasal obstruction which wakes them at night, this side-effect can be helpful, but during the day the sedation makes life 'flat' and can be dangerous if the patient has to drive or use machinery. The effects are exacerbated when the patient drinks alcohol and he should be warned against this.

Combinations of antihistamines with sympathomimetic (drugs which have the side-effect of stimulating the central nervous system) are popular. Examples include Actifed (a mixture of pseudoephidrine and tripolidine), Triominic and Eskornade (which contains isopropamide, an atropine like drug). These are often helpful in reducing the rhinorrhoea and nasal congestion in the common cold. Such drugs used systemically do not produce the same problems of rebound as rhinitis medicamentosa and may be used to wean the patient off the habitual use of drops and sprays. On the other hand, pseudoephedrine is the only systemic decongestant in the 'limited list' of drugs which are available for National Health Service prescription after 1st April 1985. This drug has the drawbacks of sympathomimetic drugs (see p. 273) and as it tends to interfere with sleep, it is a poor choice for the vast majority of patients in whom the symptom of nasal obstruction is most troublesome at night.

EAR

Topical

Preparations used in the Removal of Wax

The commonest ear problem is that of wax. If this builds up to completely occlude the meatus, there is deafness and discomfort; there may be tinnitus and pain. Various proprietary drops are available for this condition; some are intended to be used as a lubricant prior to syringing, and others soften the wax and enable it to discharge spontaneously. However, some preparations contain terebinth (turpentine) which may be painful in the ear and sometimes otitis externa develops. Probably just as effective are sodium bicarbonate ear drops (which contain glycerol), warm olive oil or arachis oil. A new preparation (Exterol) of urea hydrogen peroxide in glycerin is non-antigenic, safe and can be recommended.

Topical Antibiotics—Antiseptics

Although ear infection may occur acutely, the disease is long standing in the vast majority of patients seen in ENT departments. These patients are thus likely to have medicines for prolonged periods. Because ear infections do not readily respond to drugs, patients may also have been given a variety in the hope that one will be more successful than the rest. Chemicals may penetrate epithelial surfaces, particularly if they are inflamed, and by combination with body proteins produce an antigen. A local tissue immune response may subsequently occur as the skin becomes sensitized to the drug, producing chronic eczematous changes, adding to the difficulties of successful treatment—intensive treatment over a short period is best.

If longer term treatment is required, simple safe substances should be used; these include hydrogen peroxide, white vinegar (dilute acetic acid) and spirit drops. For otitis externa, a wick moistened with a solution of steroid and an antiseptic (incorporating a fungicide or an antibiotic which cannot be given systemically) can be used for a few days where stenosis prevents toilet; generally the canal will then open up and can be cleaned more effectively. For people prone to recurrent otitis externa, particularly if their job predisposes to this (e.g. the professional diver), thorough cleansing of the ear using water from a fresh water shower followed by instillation of spirit drops can be recommended. In cases of CSOM, topical drops of antibiotic, steroid or a combination of both are useful to settle flare-ups of infection. Cleansing both for CSOM and otitis externa using hydrogen peroxide ear-drops applied liberally is safe and often effective. Where excessive otorrhoea is the main problem, powders which can be insufflated may be more effective than drops, such as acid boric and iodine powder (ABI), provided the patient is not in the small group sensitive to iodine, or povidone-iodine powder.

Systemic Antibiotics in ENT

Many of the troublesome infections of the upper respiratory tract are of viral origin, for example coryza and most cases of sore throat; these are not affected by drugs presently available (though the symptoms may be helped). Of the bacterial infections the most serious is due to the haemolytic streptococcus. This is sensitive to penicillin, and penicillin has been used prophylactically to prevent such infection in children prone to tonsillitis or in whom the infection would be particularly dangerous (e.g. those with renal or cardiac disease). The majority of infecting bacteria isolated from the ENT territory are sensitive to penicillin, though if the infection is acquired in hospital this is less likely to be the case. The role of anaerobic organisms in infections of the ears, nose and throat has only recently become widely recognized; these organisms often exist alongside aerobic ones. Fortunately, the drug metranidazole has proved effective; it is safe, has negligible side-effects, does not produce hypersensitivity in the patient nor result in the emergence of resistant strains. When given together with one of the newer penicillins it has greatly reduced the incidence of postoperative wound infection, particularly in the irradiated patient.

Systemic antibiotics generally have no place in the treatment of CSOM or in otitis externa. However, systemic antibiotics are indicated in malignant otitis externa, where diabetes is also present, or where tender regional lymph nodes or systemic symptoms indicate spread of infection.

Penicillin is generally effective in acute otitis media and acute sinusitis; the newer synthetic penicillins or erythromycin can be reserved for patients not responding, but when using antibiotics one should be conscious of the ecological hazard of the emergence of resistant strains.

Suppositories

The administration of drugs via the rectum is less popular in Britain than in some other countries; but it may be useful in ENT practice. Examples include:

1 Stemetil can be given rectally in patients who are nauseated or vomiting from vestibular disturbance.

2 Ergotamine suppositories are useful, given prophylactically, for patients prone to be woken during the night with migrainous neuralgia: they are inserted before the patient goes to sleep.

3   Metranidazole suppositories may be given in the early post-operative period following major head and neck surgery when the drug cannot be given orally.

4   Aminophylline suppositories may be given with the pre-medication to patients subject to asthma.

Recommended for Reference

Ballantyne J. & Groves J. (1978) *A Synopsis of Otolaryngology*, 3rd edn. John Wright & Sons, Bristol.

Ballantyne J. & Groves J. (1979) *Scott-Brown's Diseases of the Ear, Nose and Throat*, 4th edn. Butterworth, London.

Beagley H. A. & Barnard S. (1982) *Manual of Audiometric Techniques*. Oxford University Press.

Bull T. R. (1974) *A Colour Atlas of ENT*. Wolfe Medical Publications, London.

Hall I. S. & Colman B. H. (1981) *Diseases of the Nose, Throat and Ear*, 12th edn. Churchill Livingstone, Edinburgh.

Last R. J. (1978) *Anatomy Regional and Applied*, 6th edn. Churchill Livingstone, Edinburgh.

Maran A. G. D. & Stell P. (1978) *Head and Neck Surgery*, 2nd edn. Heinemann, London.

Maran A. G. D. & Stell P. (1979) *Clinical Ototlaryngology*. Blackwell Scientific, Oxford.

Mawson S. R. & Ludman H. (1979) *Diseases of the Ear*, 4th edn. Edward Arnold, London.

Morrison J. D., Mirakhur R. K. & Craig H. J. L. (1985) *Anaesthesia for Eye, Ear, Nose and Throat Surgery*, 2nd edn. Churchill Livingstone, Edinburgh.

Romanes G. J. (1979) *Cunningham Textbook of Anatomy, Vol. 3: The Head, Neck and Brain*. Oxford University Press.

Shaheen, O. H. (1984) *Problems in Head and Neck Surgery*. Balliere Tindall, London.

Further Reading

Ballantyne J. & Martin J. A. M. (1984) *Deafness*, 4th edn. Churchill Livingstone, Edinburgh.

Bloom F. (1978) *Our Deaf Children into the 80s*. Gresham Publications, London.

Boore J. (1978) *Prescription for Recovery*. The Royal College of Nursing, London.

Bridge W. & Macleod Clark J. (1981) *Communication in Nursing Care*. H.M. & M., Aylesbury.

Bull T. & Cook J. (1976) *Speech Therapy and ENT Surgery*. Blackwell Scientific, Oxford.

Hayward J. (1975) *Information—A Prescription Against Pain*. The Royal College of Nursing, London.

Hunt J. & Marks-Maran D. (1980) *Nursing Care Plans. The Nursing Process at Work*. H.M. & M., Aylesbury.

Jolly J. (1981) *The Other Side of Paediatrics*. Macmillan, London.

Lamberton R. (1981) *Care of the Dying*. Pelican Books, Middlesex.

Maram A. G. D. (1983) *Otorhinolaryngology*. Volume 4, The New Medicine Series. MTP Press Ltd, Lancaster.

Piff C. (1985) *Let's Face It*. Victor Gollancz, London.

Sofaer B. (1984) *Pain; a Handbook for Nurses*. Harper & Row, London.

Stockwell F. (1981) *The Unpopular Patient*. Croom Helm, London.

Reed M. (1984) *Educating Hearing Impaired Children*. Open University Press.

Index

Page numbers in italics refer to illustrations